"Resounding with these accelerated times Brett Bevell reveals a quantum approach to practicing an age-old healing art, applying the power of intent to merge with Divine Consciousness. Within Reiki, as also with shamanism, our intentions – and our openness to the moment – are everything. *New Reiki Software for Diving Living* is an exciting guidebook for energy workers, also encouraging each of us to explore fresh possibilities for working with the Universal Life Force Energy – and for living."
Llyn Roberts, the award winning author of *Shapeshifting into Higher Consciousness*, and co-author of *Shamanic Reiki*. www.LlynRoberts.com and www.EarthWisdomCircle.org

"Brett Bevell is an extraordinary healer and I can only hope he spreads the magic of his Reiki theories far and wide. We can all use some of what he's got!"
Krista Vernoff, Emmy-nominated Screenwriter/Executive Producer for *Grey's Anatomy* & HBO's *Shameless*. Co-Author of *The Game On! Diet*.

"As a dancer, I have always been sensitive to energy and have responded well to energetic healing. Brett's work is magical and has helped me pass through emotional obstacles with ease and grace."
Carrie Ann Inaba, Judge on ABC's *Dancing with the Stars*; Actress & Choreographer; Dizzy Feet Foundation Co-founder; Founder, The Carrie Ann Inaba Animal Project.

New Reiki Software for Divine Living

An Energetic Embodiment
of Divine Grace

New Reiki
Software for
Divine Living

An Energetic Embodiment
of Divine Grace

Brett Bevell

AYNI
BOOKS

Winchester, UK
Washington, USA

First published by Ayni Books, 2013
Ayni Books is an imprint of John Hunt Publishing Ltd., Laurel House, Station Approach,
Alresford, Hants, SO24 9JH, UK
office1@jhpbooks.net
www.johnhuntpublishing.com
www.ayni-books.com

For distributor details and how to order please visit the 'Ordering' section on our website.

Text copyright: Brett Bevell 2013

ISBN: 978 1 78279 004 4

A CIP catalogue record for this book is available from the British Library.

Design: Stuart Davies

Printed and bound by CPI Group (UK) Ltd, Croydon, CR0 4YY

We operate a distinctive and ethical publishing philosophy in all
areas of our business, from our global network of authors to
production and worldwide distribution.

CONTENTS

For Helema Kadir, and all the people of the world working for peace.

Acknowledgements

I owe gratitude to all the Reiki teachers who came before me, as well as my Reiki guides, including Mother Mary, Lady of the Lake, Reiki's founding teacher Mikao Usui, the angels of Reiki, Jesus, Merlin, Pan and all the myriad teachers on the spiritual plane who have assisted me in bringing forth this new information about Reiki. Also, I need to acknowledge the Omega Institute and all of those who have supported the new and cutting edge energy healing classes I have offered there, including Lois Guarino, Britta Larsen, Carol Donahoe, Brian Schorn, Jean LaPlante, Kathy Fitzgerald, plus the many graduates of the Omega Institute Peace Guild from 2003 through to the present day. And, finally, I must acknowledge the woman who has kept me grounded through all of my energetic experiments, my dear wife Helema. She has been the firm ground that has allowed me to understand what it means to fly and return home. Without her, it is likely I would always be exploring the outer limits of my own magical consciousness, never taking the time to sit down and write this book.

Introduction

Imagine, if you will, being like a child where God has given you a ball of sacred light that lives near your heart. Inside of this ball exists the magic of Divine grace as a sacred light that can shine inner peace, calm, emotional healing, and physical wellness to anyone. Imagine then if you will that this ball of light already exists, and that you do not need to be a child to inherit this gift. All you need is the heart of a child, a willingness to suspend your inner cynic, and to let go into the realm of play.

The contents of this book explores that sacred ball of light, a profound gift I call Mikao Usui's Reiki Crystal of Awakening which came to me while traveling in Laos during January 2007. This Reiki crystal will also be gifted to you in the following pages. As you read this book, you engage a Divine energy transmission sent through these pages that revolutionizes Reiki as an energy healing system. This transmission makes it possible for even the novice Reiki student to perform Reiki treatments previously considered far beyond the norm of what even the most advanced Reiki Master teachers could do. Not only does this book offer a dynamic and radical view of what is possible with Reiki, but it does so in a way that dramatically simplifies the entire Reiki system. With the information in this book, it is now possible to perform a deep and powerful Reiki treatment without the long sequence of hand positions that has been traditionally taught to Reiki initiates. Also, with this new information it is now possible to send a Reiki treatment across space and time without having to ever memorize or use any Reiki symbols. And, perhaps most importantly, the entire system of degrees within Reiki is eliminated, making it a truly democratic and egalitarian energy healing system. In this new Reiki system even a brand-new Reiki student is capable of initiating others as Reiki practitioners.

I know with great certainty that some may find this new Reiki system frightening, as is often the case when our view of something comforting and familiar is changed. Yet it is for the greater good that I offer this book to the world.

My wish and hope is that the information in this book is so easy to learn, and so captivating to use, that the energy of Reiki will become readily available for all humankind. I envision a day when it is as common for parents to teach Reiki to their children as it is for them to show their children how to ride bicycles. The potential exists for us all to have this sacred ball of light from God, this embodiment of Divine grace in the form of this Reiki crystal. All we need to do is lift our hearts to be innocent and open, to accept this gift with the playful curiosity of a young child.

If you chose to step forward into the work of this book be ready for your life to change, and most importantly be ready to play with the Divine.

Chapter I

The Evolution of Reiki

Reiki is considered by many to be the world's most popular form of energy healing, and its origins can be traced to a Japanese mystic named Mikao Usui, who lived from 1865 to 1926. There are many stories about Mikao Usui, some referring to him as a Christian minister and others referring to him as a Buddhist monk. However, what I find important in all the stories about him is that he was a man who surrendered his ego, his life, and his spiritual process to the Divine, often using the time-honored method of fasting and prayer on his quest to rediscover the ancient spiritual healing abilities mentioned in sacred scriptures. Through this deep level of surrender, Usui was able to access this amazingly healing energy he called Reiki, a term which translates from Japanese as *Universal Life Force*.

Reiki was brought to the United States shortly before World War Two by a Japanese-American Reiki master named Hawayo Takata. Takata taught twenty-two Reiki masters over the course of her life, and Reiki has grown exponentially ever since. Today, Reiki can be found in some of the world's more progressive hospitals, and continues to evolve as an energy healing system with many branches, schools and varied ways of teaching. There are members of the Reiki Alliance who stay very close to the Reiki teachings brought to America by Takata. There is the International Center for Reiki Training in Michigan, founded by William Rand, a teacher who has done a great deal of work to make Reiki more accessible to the general public. One can also find many independent Reiki teachers who are not aligned with any particular school, but who offer their wisdom with an open heart and lead workshops in their communities to continue spreading this sacred light.

Reiki has changed my own life in amazing ways. As one who underwent a very difficult childhood and spent the first twenty years of my life extremely shy and depressed, Reiki has helped me transform and move beyond my own childhood trauma to such a degree that my life is now very celebratory, filled with abundance and love. I have taught Reiki to thousands of students, and I often receive e-mails and messages from people around the world who repeatedly confirm the miracle that Reiki has to offer: an energy healing form that is an embodiment of Divine grace, which can at times guide people out of the most troubled circumstances. These circumstances can sometimes be an issue related to physical health, but often can just as likely be about transforming a troubled relationship, overcoming depression, discovering one's life calling, creating harmony at work, and so forth.

I do not claim to know everything there is to know about Reiki. For it is a vast field with many amazing teachers. One thing I do know from my own experience with Reiki is that even though it is an elegant and beautiful system of energy healing, it can also at times intimidate those who need it most. This intimidation seems to come from several areas with respect to Reiki training. Some students forget the many hand positions and their sequencing as often taught during Reiki first degree training, and thus refrain from actually using Reiki on themselves or others after their training. Others may go on to second degree Reiki training, but then cannot fully remember the Reiki symbols, some of which can be quite complex to learn. Others get confused about techniques for sending a Reiki treatment at a distance. Then there are those who are dedicated Reiki practitioners who make it all the way through Reiki Master training, who then never teach Reiki to even one student because they are too intimidated by the Reiki initiation process. Reiki is amazing, and has the capacity to benefit each of us, and all of humanity. Yet it can only reach the greatest numbers if it is accessible and user friendly to all.

I must confess that, even though I have a reputation for wanting to make Reiki more democratic and more readily available to people, I was probably too arrogant in my own Reiki teachings for many years. If a student couldn't learn the hand positions, I considered them lazy. If a second degree student didn't fully know the Reiki symbols, I thought they were not a truly dedicated student. If I met a Reiki Master who never taught others because they were intimidated by the process, I was often a little dismissive and labeled them in my mind as somehow incompetent. Instead of seeing them with compassion and acknowledging that the road to healing and grace can be difficult enough without the added burden of feeling like a failed teacher of a complex system. Even though as a Reiki Master author I was often considered on the cutting edge of my field, I must admit that in many ways I had yet to fully know the deepest teaching of Reiki: which is that Reiki is a gift from the Divine to all humanity, not something anyone should have to learn tricks to perform. We are not circus animals and Reiki should not be considered a kind of reward or prize only to be made available to those who have the best memory, or who are the least intimidated.

I have the greatest reverence for the Reiki system as it is taught traditionally. I enjoy using the sacred Reiki symbols and giving treatments that require me to access the sequence of many Reiki hand positions. I love seeing when a student can draw the symbols without my assistance. I feel great when seeing a room of students all gently flowing this fabulous energy from their hands, and all feeling confident in their ability to offer a Reiki treatment. Yet I know that this complexity which has evolved around Reiki is not the heart of Reiki itself. The heart of Reiki is simply an energetic embodiment of Divine grace, and that is something which should be available to all, not simply those who are the most adept at learning.

Since my first exposure to Reiki I have known that Reiki is evolving. It is not a stagnant system as some might teach it to be, but is one which dances with our consciousness as we grow in our capacity to understand the universe and the Divine. This knowing has been with me since my first day of being initiated into Reiki, and has given me the gift of seeing things that are possible within the Reiki system which may not be considered as possible by others. I often talk to my Reiki guides and ask to be shown new symbols and new techniques. I test what I am shown, often demanding for repeated results to confirm a technique works before I pass it on as a teaching to my students. When I was finishing the final chapters of my previous Reiki book, *Reiki for Spiritual Healing* (Crossing Press, 2009), I asked my guides if there was anything new to Reiki that could add to the process of spiritual awakening, since the theme of using Reiki for spiritual awakening was the core teaching of the book. When I asked this question, sitting at my computer in my office, I felt an opening in my heart. The opening was huge and filled with Reiki light, and felt to me like it was coming directly from the spirit of the late Mikao Usui, who is the founding teacher of Reiki. This ball of Reiki light opened my heart so dramatically, that I then asked it to send Reiki energy out to energetically bathe all readers who would eventually read *Reiki for Spiritual Healing* at the time of their reading the book. Even though the energy transmissions, which are sent to all who read *Reiki for Spiritual Healing*, were coming from this ball of Reiki light, I was told by my guides that my understanding of this ball of Reiki light was still far too limited to actually teach it to others. So, I left out any mention of it in that book, waiting until the time was right and my understanding deep enough to make the teachings worthy.

I have since been experimenting with this ball of Reiki light for several years, and see that not only is it a higher and more intense vibration of Reiki energy than most Reiki symbols can access, but that it is an actual energy crystal made of Reiki light, imbued with Divine intelligence, guided and overseen by the spirit of Mikao Usui. I call this Reiki energy crystal *Mikao Usui's Reiki Crystal of Awakening*.

At first I was unaware that this crystal held the ability to unify the entire Reiki system into one level of teaching. I simply knew the crystal was powerful and offered immense healing capacity. I taught a few students, mostly during workshops I offered at Omega Institute titled *Reiki & the Magic of Awakening*. Students seemed to love the energy and healing that this new Reiki tool offered, and yet I as the teacher was still missing a big part of what this crystal was about. It has only been very recently, after October of 2011 when I taught a Reiki Master workshop at Omega Institute, that I began to see the immense capacity of that this Reiki crystal offers. Although the workshop in October 2011 was a traditional Reiki Master training, during many of the meditations held that week I often saw and felt the presence of Mother Mary, who is one of my strongest Reiki guides. The spirit of Mother Mary informed me that another book on Reiki was going to be downloaded to me in the near future, and that is the book you now hold in your hands.

Should you decide to read onwards through the following chapters you will be empowered to this new Reiki crystal, which is a crystal of Divine Reiki light imbued with Divine intelligence. It has the capacity to send Reiki at a distance, offer Reiki empowerments to others, and even focus Reiki during a treatment to specific systems within the body, such as the nervous system or circulatory system. It simplifies Reiki in such a profound way that anyone can learn it, and can use it effectively. I am not saying that there is no longer any reason to be trained in the various levels of Reiki, or to abandon the system of powerful Reiki symbols. However, I am saying that there is now a much simpler road to get to those same healing destinations, while still using the energy of Reiki in a form which is more powerful than many of the more cumbersome and complicated techniques of the past.

I hope you will step forward with me on this journey, one which holds the promise of making Reiki available to all, even to those who are impatient, those who are self-critical, those who might have a hard time learning the complexities of Reiki symbols and hand positions, but who are no less deserving of this energetic form of Divine grace called Reiki.

Chapter 2

Mikao Usui's Reiki Crystal of Awakening

Mikao Usui's Reiki Crystal of Awakening is the most advanced Reiki tool I have ever experienced or known. It works from a place of Divine grace and is guided by Divine intelligence. Yet because it is imbued with this deep sense of Divine grace, it is full of grace, or in other words graceful. It is elegant and serene in all of its functions. Mikao Usui's Reiki Crystal of Awakening is an energetic embodiment of all Reiki teachings, all Reiki possibilities, all Reiki lineages. It is all inclusive of all Reiki symbols, and evolves with human consciousness so that as new Reiki possibilities emerge, they are made immediately available through this amazing crystal.

How this crystal works is also amazingly simple: it runs by intention. If you intend the crystal to send Reiki to your stomach, it will. If you intend it to send Reiki to your liver, it will send Reiki to your liver. If you ask for it to send a treatment for a specific period of minutes, it will send Reiki for that specific amount of time. All that is required of the practitioner is to clearly focus their intention and ask the Reiki crystal to perform the requested function.

This crystal can also perform more than one function simultaneously, such as sending Reiki to your nervous system while also sending Reiki to an issue in your past that might be the cause of a specific nervous disorder. Or sending Reiki to your digestive system while also sending Reiki to a meal you had earlier in the day which may be the cause of an upset stomach. The crystal is literally programmed by your own thoughts or vocal command, and guided by Divine intelligence, so that no harm can come from using the crystal.

If you are someone who is already a trained Reiki practitioner who enjoys sending Reiki treatments to others, or even a Reiki novice, you can now use this crystal to send Reiki treatments to numerous people simultaneously, again by simply intending it to happen. Other things you can do with the crystal include programming an entire treatment for yourself, setting the intention of the specific areas of the body where the Reiki energy will flow, how long for each area, while also including any specific sequence of how the energy might flow. Then once you have set that intention you simply relax and enjoy the treatment.

All of this may seem far too radical for those who have been trained in Reiki, who are used to having to incorporate the Reiki symbols and specific hand positions in order to attain certain results. Yet this new Reiki crystal is truly a gift from the Divine, an expression of Reiki as Divine grace, which does not require our wisdom, our intellect, or any expertise to be welcomed by its capacity to heal and change our lives. Once you have been empowered with this Reiki crystal you can use the practice sessions in order to fully understand how easily this new Reiki system works.

The empowerment, which is made available in the following chapter, will create an energetic Reiki crystal located in the area near the front of the middle of your chest, a few inches in front of your sternum. For those who are familiar with the Indian system of seven chakras of the human energy body, this Reiki crystal will exist in the area in front of the heart chakra. However, if you are unfamiliar with the chakra system, it is not necessary for you to have any understanding of that energy system in order to use Mikao Usui's Reiki Crystal of Awakening. Simply know that once empowered you will have an energetic crystal made of Divine Reiki light, about the size of a golf ball, existing a few inches in front of the middle of your chest. You will most likely not be able to feel the presence of this Reiki crystal, except for when you are using it.

The way I like to think of this Reiki crystal is as a computer chip that is part of a Divine Reiki computer, capable of sending Reiki to any place at any point in time and space. Once you input your intention into this computer, through your visualization, your words, or through thought, then the Reiki crystal activates Reiki to flow as you intended it. It is very easy, very simple, once you become familiar with the process. And for those who also prefer the human touch aspect of Reiki, as it has been taught for generations in traditional first degree Reiki training, you will also have the ability to use the Reiki crystal to make Reiki flow directly out of your hands. For those who are already trained as Reiki Masters, you will find that the Reiki crystal can also perform functions previously unheard of in the Reiki system, which will be more thoroughly explained in later chapters. Mikao Usui's Reiki Crystal of Awakening offers something positive for all, regardless of your level of previous Reiki training or other energy healing experience.

The following chapter holds the ability to radically change your life for the better, should you decide to embrace the energetic empowerment which will give you your own personal version of Mikao Usui's Reiki Crystal of Awakening. In my previous Reiki books I suggested a specific number of hours one might offer as community service as their energy exchange for the Reiki initiations offered in those books, such as offering Reiki to the sick or elderly, or sending Reiki to help heal the Earth. Yet do to the unique and profound nature of Mikao Usui's Reiki Crystal of Awakening, and that it is truly an energetic embodiment of Divine grace, my guidance tells me that no energy exchange is required for those Reiki students, new or experienced, who wish to be initiated to this new form of Reiki. It, like grace, is truly a gift from the Divine, bestowed on any who wish to receive it. However, should you wish to give thanks to the Divine by offering some form of spiritual service to your community in return, that is also acceptable and honorable. That service can be in the form of volunteering time for a worthy cause, giving money to charity, or offering your new Reiki skills for several hours to those who need it free of charge. Please know this energy exchange is not required and should only happen if you truly feel moved to offer it, not from any false sense of obligation.

The following chapter offers an energy empowerment that is embedded into the text. Once you begin reading it, the empowerment for Mikao Usui's Reiki Crystal of Awakening will begin to build in your energy system. By the time you have finished reading the following chapter, that energy transmission will be complete, and you will be fully empowered to this new form of Reiki, which is simple, easy to use, and as powerful as any form of Reiki presently on the planet. Should you wish to mark the sacredness of the occasion, you may want to take a ritual bath with a pinch of sea salt in the bath to cleanse your aura or energy field. You might also want to light a candle to the Divine, by whatever name you call God or Goddess. Maybe you will want to simply acknowledge that each breath and each moment in this journey called life is sacred, and continue reading without doing anything to mark the specialness of this occasion. Either way is fine and good, just as Divine grace can find us in the most sacred temples, and can also find us in the supermarket. The only thing that matters is to ask for it and embrace it with an open heart.

Please know, however, that once you become empowered to this new form of Reiki, it will raise your overall energy vibration, even if you are already a Reiki Master. This change on your energy vibration will also often result in life changes such as a shift in your career, getting into or out of a relationship, finding new friends and releasing old friendships that no longer serve your highest good. You may even sometimes experience cravings for new types of food that may result in an entirely new diet. Know as well that whatever these changes may be, they are for the highest good. In some instances those changes may not always be comfortable or easy. Be ready for the ride you are about to embark upon once you read the following chapter. Even if you never use the techniques taught in this book, if you accept the empowerment in the following chapter it is bound to change your life for the better, simply by raising your overall energy vibration to a new level.

Chapter 3

Becoming Attuned to Mikao Usui's Reiki Crystal of Awakening

This book is sending you a Divine and powerful new form of Reiki called Mikao Usui's Reiki Crystal of Awakening. As you read this text, this new form of Reiki is being sent through these words. This book is sending a Reiki healing transmission which will continue for as long as you are reading this chapter. Once you complete reading the text of this chapter, reading it once through from start to finish, you will be fully empowered with Mikao Usui's Reiki Crystal of Awakening. Please know that this healing power does not come from the author of this book. This is an example of Divine grace in energetic form. This is a gift from that which is Pure Love. This is a gift from that Which is All. Even if you are someone who does not feel energy healing, please continue reading.

What is happening now as you read is what will happen when you yourself decide to empower others in this new form of Reiki healing. A small and yet infinite piece of Mikao Usui's Reiki Crystal of Awakening is moving out to you now. Imagine that this book contains a small sun within it. Imagine that sun is made of Reiki light. Now imagine that small sun of Reiki light is shooting out from this book, like a solar flare, and reaching into your heart. Once it touches your heart chakra, or the area a few inches in front of the middle of your chest, it is there developing like a photograph, creating an image of itself, like a new sun made of Reiki light. And know that this sun of Reiki light radiating from the center of your chest is actually an energy crystal which can react to, and be moved by, your own thoughts. It is still developing and not yet fully formed, but it will be fully formed by the time you complete reading this chapter.

Play with this Divine crystal of Reiki light by imagining your thoughts moving down into it and giving it a command. As long as the command is for the highest good, the Reiki crystal will send Reiki as you have requested. Begin first by sending your thoughts into this Reiki crystal, which you can imagine as made out of pure white light in the area a few inches in front of the middle of your chest. Ask this Reiki crystal to send you Reiki, asking either out loud by using your voice, or by simply asking with your mind. Ask this Reiki crystal to now send Reiki to your entire nervous system for the next five minutes. Allow your being to be filled with this Divine light, this gift, this energetic form of Divine grace.

Know that Mikao Usui's Reiki Crystal of Awakening is almost fully formed now in your own energy system. That small piece of infinite Reiki light, which came from the infinite Reiki light embedded into the text of this book, has crystalized with your own thought process. It will now move Reiki according to your own thoughts, as long as those thoughts are for the highest good.

Breathe now, and feel the Reiki crystal presence that was coming from this book be fully downloaded into your own energy system. Ask for this Reiki crystal to send Reiki to your mind. Feel the Reiki as it flows to you, out from the Reiki crystal in the center of your chest so that this light is bathing your thoughts.

Know that you cannot do this incorrectly. There is no right or wrong way to do this. This is an energetic gift from the Divine, and once you complete reading this text, regardless of how well you follow the instructions of the text, you will be empowered to Mikao Usui's Reiki Crystal of Awakening simply by the act of reading this full text.

Take another breath, as the Reiki crystal in this book is now sending Reiki energy into your breath. Pull this energy into your lungs and imagine that with each breath you are pulling more and more Reiki light into this new Reiki crystal that now exists a few inches in front of the center of your chest, like a radiant ball of Divine Reiki light.

Allow yourself to sigh if you feel the need. As many often do at this point in the transmission. Now, press your hands together, and simply ask with your intentions that the Reiki crystal, which is now fully functioning in your own energy system, send Reiki through both of your hands. Continue pressing your hands together, and simply notice what you feel. You may feel an intense amount of heat or strong vibration between your hands, or you may feel nothing at all. Please know each of us has their own level of sensitivity to energy healing, and that the real impact is not about feeling the energy, but about healing ourselves and changing our lives for the better.

Know that you are now fully empowered to Mikao Usui's Reiki Crystal of Awakening. You can now send Reiki simply by asking the crystal to send it for you. Know that an intense level of Reiki can also now flow out of your hands, flowing directly from the Reiki crystal upon your intention through your hands into anything you touch. Also if you are a Reiki novice, you now have a new Reiki energetic tool that is extremely powerful and yet elegant to use. If you are one who has had previous Reiki experience, and perhaps are even a fully trained Reiki Master, know that you now have a new Reiki tool which compliments all the Reiki skills you have learned in the past, and which elevates them to an even higher level of ability.

Give thanks in whatever form you wish, to those who have given us the gift of Reiki at this appointed time. Give thanks to the Divine, by whatever name you wish to use for the Divine. Give thanks to the angels and spirits that oversee Reiki. Give thanks to Mikao Usui and all the Reiki teachers who came after him. You are now fully empowered to Mikao Usui's Reiki Crystal of Awakening. Celebrate, or relax. Laugh or weep tears of joy. Be still with wisdom, or ecstatic with excitement. And know regardless of your own reaction to reading this text that you now have hardwired into your energetic system an energetic embodiment of Divine grace in the form of Reiki. It is permanent. It can never be taken from you. It does not come from the author of this book. This gift is directly from the Divine.

Chapter 4

The Basic Reiki Crystal Self Treatment

You are now empowered to Mikao Usui's Reiki Crystal of Awakening, which is an elegant, powerful, and yet simple form of Reiki. To perform a self treatment using this new form of Reiki, begin by knowing there are only three primary hand positions: hands on the head, hands on the heart or chest area, and hands on the stomach or lower belly. Exact placement is unnecessary, so your primary obligation is to let comfort be your guide in how you approximate each hand placement.

Begin the Reiki crystal self treatment by first placing your hands anywhere you wish on your head. You may cradle the back of your head with your fingers interlaced. You may cover your eyes with one hand over each eye. You can rest your hands over the sides of your face. Or, you might wish to gently rest both palms on the top of your head. Do whatever variation makes you comfortable. All that is important is that your hands be touching your head.

Once your hands are touching your head, intend the Reiki crystal to flow Reiki directly out of your hands. You may notice a tingling sensation or heat being generated by your hands as you do this. Or, you may not feel anything at all. Whatever your experience is, is right. There is no right or wrong for how your experience should be. Please know that some people are more sensitive to Reiki than others, but that Reiki will still work on those who do not necessarily feel it. The true test of your experience should be in seeing how your mental, emotional and physical wellness improves with repeated use of Reiki.

Hold your hands on your head in a comfortable position for approximately ten minutes. Allow the Reiki energy to radiate all through your head, through the muscles of your face, into the inner ear, the sinus cavities, into your eyes, the bones of your skull, and into your brain. The power of Mikao Usui's Reiki Crystal of Awakening allows the Reiki practitioner to be less exact in their hand placement, and yet still bathe an entire region of their body with Reiki light. So, as long as you place your hands on some part of your head, your entire head will receive a deep and powerful Reiki healing within the ten-minute period of time.

Once the ten-minute session on your head is complete, then gently move your hands down to the region of your chest. You can place your hands over the region of your heart, your lungs, one hand over each breast, or any variation that feels comfortable to you. Hold your hands in the area of your chest for ten minutes, while intending or asking that the Reiki crystal send Reiki through your hands into the area of your chest. Allow the Reiki energy to radiate through all the important organs of your chest, into your heart, into your lungs, into the bones of your sternum and into your ribs and the connective tissue around all of these. The power of Mikao Usui's Reiki Crystal of Awakening will bathe all of your chest with an intense vibration of Reiki energy, so again exact placement of your hands is not important, as long as they are somewhere in the area of your chest. Simply hold the hand placement for approximately ten minutes, and allow this simple but powerful form of Reiki healing to run its course.

After the ten-minute session on the area of your chest is complete, move your hands gently to your belly. Then intend the Reiki crystal flow Reiki through your hands into the area of your belly. Allow the Reiki energy to flow into your stomach, your intestines, your liver, gallbladder, colon, all the important muscles and connective tissue in that area of your body. Again, since the higher and more intense vibration of Mikao Usui's Reiki Crystal of Awakening has a deeper effect on that entire region of your body, it is not important for your hand placement to be exact or specific. Trust in the flow of Divine energy, and then simply surrender. Hold the hand placement in the area of your belly for approximately ten minutes, and then when it feels like enough time has passed, rest your hands by your sides, or leave them comfortably placed on your belly or chest, whichever is most comfortable.

Now, intend that Mikao Usui's Reiki Crystal of Awakening send your entire body a Reiki treatment for integration. All that you need to do is intend this to happen, and it will. If you wish, you can imagine seeing the Reiki crystal in front of the center of your chest, and then intend or imagine your thoughts going into it, programming the crystal with the intention that it run an integrating form of Reiki light on you until you are perfectly integrated from the treatment. It is not necessary to use any of the traditional Reiki symbols, nor any of the Reiki grids mentioned in my book *Reiki for Spiritual Healing* (Crossing Press, 2009). Since the Reiki crystal is guided by Divine intelligence, it will know how long to send this energy for the perfect level of integration. Normally, this will last only a few minutes.

When you have completed your first self treatment, give thanks to yourself for being a vessel of the Reiki energy. Give thanks to your Reiki guides. And give thanks to Mikao Usui and those Reiki teachers who came after him.

Chapter 5

The Advanced Reiki Crystal Self Treatment

The Reiki treatment in the previous chapter is intentionally simple, and yet also very powerful. It functions as a stand-alone treatment, and in itself will be enough for many people who want a simple and easy technique to make Reiki a part of their daily lives. Yet for those who want to add an even deeper level of healing, there is a process of using mental focus in alignment with the crystal to intend that Mikao Usui's Reiki Crystal of Awakening send Reiki in ways that will compliment the treatment from the previous chapter.

Remember, the Reiki crystal that has been created in your energy system is also linked to your own thoughts and ability to visualize, and actually requires your own mental participation in order to become fully functional. The Reiki crystal is not just an energetic device added to your own energy system, but is a ball of Reiki light that is crystalized with your own consciousness and Divine consciousness merging to be its guide. You can even think of this Reiki crystal as being a nexus point where your own consciousness and Divine consciousness can meet, which is the subject for even deeper Reiki meditations found in the later chapters of this book.

Let's begin with some very simple exercises to train your mind in how to use this Reiki crystal as a healing tool. Do this first without using any of the three hand positions mentioned in the previous chapter, though later you can add hand positions for a deeper and more layered Reiki treatment. So, begin with a very easy self treatment using only the Reiki crystal.

Start by bringing the attention of your consciousness to your Reiki crystal. If you see it, you may experience this crystal as a ball of white or even translucent light in the area a few inches in front of the middle of your chest. If you are not one who sees energy, you may simply imagine seeing this crystal. Since the process of using the crystal works by intention, actually seeing it is not as important as simply focusing your mental attention on the crystal.

Now that your mental attention is on the crystal, imagine your thoughts actually going into the crystal to program it with the intention that Reiki flow through your entire body for five minutes, or gently whisper this intention to the crystal with your voice. Either technique will activate Reiki energy to flow from the crystal through your entire body for five minutes. Although you could intend it to be a longer treatment, keep the treatment to five minutes so that you can practice and continue working with this process as outlined in this chapter. Once you have programmed the crystal with your thoughts, simply relax and enjoy the mini Reiki treatment, knowing you can resume reading this chapter once the treatment has ended.

You have now hopefully experienced how simple and easy it is to use Mikao Usui's Reiki Crystal of Awakening for a short five-minute treatment. This technique is incredibly simple, and yet can have many variations. Let's play with the technique of using the crystal to focus Reiki now on a specific organ. As before, bring your mental attention on to the Reiki crystal, either by seeing it or imagining that you see it. Once your mental attention is on the crystal, tell it with your mind or your voice to now send a five-minute Reiki treatment to your liver. Imagine your thoughts actually going into the crystal to program it with your intention, or whisper the instructions to the Reiki crystal as if speaking to a friend. Upon making this request to the Reiki crystal, the crystal will begin sending Reiki to your liver. There is no need to use Reiki symbols for this sending to occur. Just focus your mental intention into the crystal, or use a gentle whisper, then relax and enjoy the treatment.

You can continue practicing this process to send Reiki to any specific organ in your body. All that is required is that you focus your mental attention on to the crystal, then imagine your thoughts going into the crystal to program it with your intention or speak gently your specific instructions to the Reiki crystal as if you were speaking to a friend. Remember, the Reiki crystal is imbued with Divine intelligence so it can hear what you think as well as what you say. Try this technique to send Reiki to a variety of organs just to get the practice. Use the crystal to send Reiki to your stomach, intestines, lungs, heart, brain, or even areas of your body that are difficult to reach such as your feet or knees. Practice for several minutes, using your own intuition and guidance to decide where you would like the Reiki crystal to send a short treatment. It will only take a few times practicing this technique to understand how easy and effective it can be.

Now that you understand how easy it is to use the Reiki crystal, combine this wisdom with the three hand positions used in Chapter Four. This is still a very easy Reiki treatment, but will be at a deeper level than if you used only the hand positions themselves.

Begin by placing your hands on your head wherever is comfortable. As you do this, simply intend that Reiki from the Reiki crystal will flow directly through your hands. Again, due to the power of this new form of Reiki, the hand position treatment by itself is quite deep and sufficient. But now you can take this treatment to an even deeper level of healing by adding specific requests into the Reiki crystal as the healing continues.

Once your hands are placed on your head and Reiki is flowing, bring your awareness to the Reiki crystal and intend with your thoughts that the Reiki crystal send the following Reiki treatment sequence. Know that you can program this full sequence into the crystal and that the crystal itself will perform these Reiki functions. If sending this sequence through your thoughts seems too difficult, you can simply speak the command out loud and the Reiki crystal will follow the exact sequence you have programmed into it through your speech. You can use speech or mental intention, whichever is easier and more comfortable for you. Please either think the following words, or say them aloud:

Mikao Usui's Reiki Crystal of Awakening
send the following Reiki treatment sequence:
five minutes of Reiki to my brain and entire nervous system,
followed by five minutes of Reiki to my lungs and respiratory system,
followed by five minutes of Reiki to my heart, blood and entire circulatory system,
followed by five minutes of Reiki to my stomach and digestive system,
followed by five minutes of Reiki to my skin, muscles and skeletal system,
followed by five minutes of integration Reiki to my entire being.

In my books *The Reiki Magic Guide to Self-Attunement* (Crossing Press, 2007) and *Reiki for Spiritual Healing*, there are Reiki chants that involve the Higher Self which often require blowing three times at the end of each chant. However, since this work does not involve or require sending energy to your Higher Self, all that is required is that the Reiki crystal be programmed, either through thought or speech, whichever is easier. No blowing or offering of breath at the end of the statement is required.

Once you have programmed the Reiki crystal, simply continue with the hand positions as outlined in Chapter Four. Hold the hand positions at the head for ten minutes, then the chest for ten minutes, then the belly for ten minutes. What happens in this combined layered form of treatment is that your hands are flowing Reiki from the crystal into specific regions of the body, while simultaneously the Reiki crystal itself is sending Reiki to entire systems within the body.

It is a wonderful way to deepen your experience of Reiki, and takes the healing to an advanced level previously unattainable in Reiki.

Chapter 6

Performing a Reiki Crystal Treatment on Another Person

I have known many who are trained in Reiki who never use Reiki on others because they are intimidated by the many hand positions taught as part of level one Reiki training. Although I have deep respect for the tradition of the Reiki hand position sequence, and know it creates a very nourishing energy healing for anyone who receives this form of treatment, I also believe that Reiki is evolving and that there are simpler ways of reaching the same goal.

Naturally, those who have spent their lives dedicated to learning the traditional Reiki form of hand sequence, and who have taught it and shared it with others, may find it offensive to suggest that there is an easier way. Yet, I see Reiki as a form of spiritual technology that is constantly being upgraded. To me, Mikao Usui's Reiki Crystal of Awakening is an upgrade to the entire Reiki system of healing. That being said, the example I like to use is that for many years I wrote my books on an old 1995 IBM Thinkpad laptop computer. It served my needs, and I understood how to use it without taking any advanced computer classes. It was functional and I didn't need anything else. If you are one who has been trained in traditional forms of Reiki and those forms work for you, there is no need to change what works for you if you prefer not to. I know that I myself will continue to teach traditional Reiki classes, from first degree all the way to Reiki Master level. I am not at all suggesting that we abandon Reiki tradition. However, I am inviting those who are willing to be open to new ways of accessing Reiki in the same way that I as a writer no longer use my 1995 IBM Thinkpad, because technology has advanced and can do more than it once could.

The same is true with the spiritual technology of Reiki.

The Reiki treatment in this chapter bypasses many of the traditional hand positions, and offers a new approach. My belief is that this new approach will be more inviting and simpler to use than traditional forms, and that this simpler form of Reiki will allow Reiki to become more popular, and thus touch the lives of more people than if we had only the traditional Reiki treatment to draw from.

To perform a Reiki treatment after being empowered with Mikao Usui's Reiki Crystal of Awakening, begin by asking the person what is their intention for the Reiki treatment. They might name a physical or emotional issue, a life circumstance, or they might simply ask for a Reiki treatment to relax and nourish.

Have the person then lie down on a massage table if one is available. If one is not available, then find a comfortable place for them to lie down, such as on the floor on a yoga mat, or on a sofa or couch. You as the Reiki practitioner can sit next the person in a chair, or on a pillow or cushion if the person is on the floor. Although it is also fine if you prefer to stand. Basically, do whatever makes you comfortable, and use common sense.

Once you and the person receiving the treatment are both comfortable and ready, begin by sending your intention into Mikao Usui's Reiki Crystal that it performs a Reiki wave across the aura of the person you are treating. A Reiki wave is a wave of energy that will slowly roll across the recipient's energy field, smoothing out any energetic stagnation and aligning their energetic system to be most receptive to the healing. It is similar to the Reiki process for smoothing the aura as mentioned in my book *The Reiki Magic Guide to Self-Attunement* (Crossing Press, 2007); however, much simpler to execute since Mikao Usui's Reiki Crystal of Awakening is doing the work for you.

Allow this Reiki wave to continue for several minutes. You may notice the person become calmer, or sigh as this process deepens with their energy system. After a few minutes, now invite your Reiki crystal to begin sending Reiki through your hands. Then, gently place your hands in a comfortable position on top of the person's head, and allow Reiki to flow from the Reiki crystal, through your hands, into the person's head. Know that as you hold this position, their entire head is filling up with Reiki light, moving through their sinuses, their ears, their facial muscles. The power of Mikao Usui's Reiki Crystal generates so much energy that the exact placement of hands on these specific areas is unnecessary. As long as you maintain your hands on the top of the recipient's head, these areas will all receive a sufficient amount of Reiki for a very deep healing.

Once the energy begins to flow out of your hands and into the person's head, you can then program the Reiki crystal to send a thirty-minute treatment on any issue named prior to the session. For example, if a person asked that the goal of the session be for mental or emotional healing, all you would need to do is bring your attention to the Reiki crystal at the center of your chest, then ask that it run a thirty-minute treatment on the person for mental or emotional healing. There is no need for you to have knowledge of or to have studied the traditional Reiki symbol for mental or emotional healing. Again, since the Reiki crystal contains all Reiki knowledge, all Reiki traditions, it knows how to activate this energy on its own. Remember, Mikao Usui's Reiki Crystal of Awakening is more than just energy, and is also infused with Divine consciousness. All you need to do is request the healing. The wisdom and Divine consciousness within the crystal does the rest.

After having named the primary goal of the treatment, simply keep your hands resting on the person's head for approximately ten minutes. Then, after ten minutes is up, gently move your hands down to the person's chest. Find a place that is comfortable to both you and the recipient for placing your hands. This can be on the upper chest between the shoulders and breasts, or on the sides of the ribs. Again, use common sense and be respectful of the person's boundaries. Once your hands are comfortably placed, intend the Reiki crystal to continue flowing Reiki from your hands so that Reiki fills the recipient's entire chest, including their heart, lungs, muscles, connective tissue etc.

Know that while you are doing this the Reiki crystal is also simultaneously still working on the primary issue named at the start of the treatment. The ability of the crystal to multitask in this manner is amazing, and will be more deeply explored in later chapters. But, for now, stay focused on the hand positions, and allowing the Reiki crystal to address the one primary issue named at the beginning of the treatment. Once you have held your hands in the area of the chest for approximately ten minutes, it is time to then move on to the next placement.

Now move your hands to the belly of the recipient; I generally like to place my hands as near as possible to their navel. But, again, simply be mindful of what seems comfortable to the person you are offering the healing to. Whether you place your hands directly near the navel, or on the sides of the belly does not need to be exact. As long as your hands are in proximity of the belly, the treatment will flow as it should. Intend that Reiki flow from the Reiki crystal, through your hands, into the person's intestines, stomach and all regions of the belly in need of Reiki. Again, since Reiki has its own Divine intelligence, you can simply place your hands in that region of the body, surrender, and let the Divine do the rest. Allow Reiki to continue to flow in this area of the belly for approximately ten minutes, and know that simultaneously Reiki is still flowing from the Reiki crystal to also address the primary issue named at the start of the treatment. Once the ten minutes ends, it is time to begin the integration portion of the treatment.

The Reiki integration light is not something that has been traditionally taught. I explore the concept thoroughly in my book *Reiki for Spiritual Healing*, and worked with the angels and devas of Reiki to create a Universal Reiki Integration Grid specifically for the purpose of creating a more integrated approach for ending a Reiki healing. The reason for integration is that often people will be energetically rewired or reconfigured during a deep treatment. Emotions move and shift. Old memories or repressed trauma may come to the surface. And though all of this is for the purpose of a greater healing, what the Reiki integration light does is help realign and reconfigure what has happened during the treatment so that the person still gains the benefits of the healing, but does so in a way that still allows them to function and go on about their day after the treatment is finished. Too often I have seen energy healers who love blasting their clients with so much energy that it can literally take days or even weeks before their client can function again as a normal human being. The purpose of Reiki integration is to make the road to healing one that is smooth and gentle.

To perform the integration aspect of the healing, simply bring your awareness to the Reiki crystal. You can actually release your hands at this point from their final placement, and allow them to rest in your own lap or at your sides. Once you have removed your hands from the person, and your awareness is fully engaged with the Reiki crystal in front of the center of your chest, simply send your thoughts or intention, or even whisper to the crystal if you wish, that it perform a Reiki integration on the recipient of the treatment. Usually, this integration will take only a few minutes. Often, you may notice during this time that the recipient, who was once in a deep sleep or trance-like state, now begins to toss and turn, or show signs of fidgeting or movement. Know that this is entirely natural. The Reiki integration will run its course in its own time. You do not need to specify the amount of time it should run. When the session is complete, you then silently thank the person for the opportunity for you to perform Reiki. You also give thanks to your guides for working with you as a Reiki healer. And then give thanks to Mikao Usui and all the Reiki teachers who came before you. Then, temporarily leave the session area and wash your hands to symbolize the session is truly complete.

Once you have engaged in a process of gratitude and hand washing, you can then return and share any insights you might have with the recipient of the treatment. Often, this is the most challenging part of the treatment. I have known many Reiki healers who unfortunately try to turn the healing into a psychic reading, which is not what it is meant to be. Also, some Reiki healers are not as accurate with psychic information as they may think they are. My recommendation is to always recommend the person drink plenty of water, and then ask them if they would like to hear anything that was sensed during the treatment. This gives the person the right to say no if they would prefer not to receive any suggestions or insights. Again, try not to turn the treatment into a psychic healing, but offer useful insights such as recommending the person be kinder to themselves, or that they take more time to relax and slow down, or eat healthier. Try to refrain from detailed analysis of their lives, their relationships or anything else that changes the function of the session from a healing into a psychic reading. Also be very mindful that unless you are a doctor you must always refrain from any attempt to diagnose an illness or disease.

Once the person leaves the session area, then ask the Reiki crystal to perform a short energy treatment of a few minutes to rebalance your own energy system.

Chapter 7

Sending Distant Treatments Using Your Reiki Crystal

Mikao Usui's Reiki Crystal of Awakening can be used to send Reiki treatments across time and space. In traditional Reiki, a person would only be able to send a distant Reiki treatment after they had training in the second degree of Reiki and had learned the distant Reiki symbol called Hon Sha Ze Sho Nen. But now, with the Divine grace that has brought forth this new Reiki crystal, it is possible to send Reiki treatments across time and space without any knowledge of the traditional second degree Reiki symbols. And, it is possible to send these treatments now, without the need for deeper levels of training and initiation.

However, the ease of this new technique for sending Reiki does not absolve one from the obligation of gaining a person's consent if you are intending to send them a Reiki treatment. Please ask someone before you send them Reiki. I have too often seen it happen in the energy healing world where new practitioners frequently fall into the poor habit of wanting to send energy healing to all their family members and friends in a dysfunctional effort to change them. Not only is this a violation of the free will of those who are not asked, but it also promotes a dysfunctional *care taking* mentality, where the practitioner avoids addressing their own issues by trying to heal everyone else's issues. That being said, I do believe there are rare instances when it is okay to assume consent, and ask for forgiveness if the consent is not given. Those cases are when there is a medical emergency. If you have a dear friend or loved one in a coma, or other medical situation where you cannot get expressed consent, then in those rare cases I feel it is better to err on the side of possibly sending Reiki when it is unwanted than to not send it at all. For years I was very strict about my guidelines in those situations, at times telling my students they should use a pendulum or other esoteric means of divination to try and find if someone's Higher Self could offer consent when their conscious self could not be asked. Yet one day during a Reiki class I was approached by woman in tears who was a member of the National Guard about to serve in the war in Afghanistan. She asked to know about the healing possibilities of using Reiki in the battlefield, and as I looked at her I knew the absurdity of me asking her to use a pendulum or other such means in the midst of war. Ever since that moment I have tried to be more compassionate in my views, and see that there are times when you may want to assume consent is given; these almost always having to do with situations of medical emergency. Other than those situations, however, you must ask the person if they wish to receive a Reiki treatment. And if they decline, then please respect their decision.

Once you gave gained permission to send someone a Reiki treatment, then ask them when they wish to receive the treatment. Know that the time when you send the treatment and the time when the other receives the treatment do not need to happen simultaneously. You can easily send a treatment forward in time, by hours, days, weeks, or months, and intend it to arrive at the appointed time requested by the recipient. However, for the purpose of simply teaching how to do a distant treatment let's assume the treatment is being sent and received in the present moment.

Begin the treatment by telling the Reiki crystal, using either your thoughts or your voice, to send Reiki to the intended person. At that point the treatment will begin. Once the treatment is initiated, intend that the crystal send Reiki to the person's entire being, and any issue they have requested you address during the treatment. As the crystal is sending Reiki, you may have a tingling sensation in the region just in front of your heart chakra, a few inches in front of the middle of your chest.

This entirely normal. Also, know you can literally program the crystal with your thoughts or voice to send Reiki for a specific amount of time. So, it is easy to just drop your consciousness down into the crystal, give it mental or vocal instructions for the entire session, and then let go of needing to focus on the session any further.

For example, if the recipient of the treatment wishes for a half-hour treatment for general stress reduction, you can simply allow your awareness to sink into the crystal and then use your thoughts or a vocal command to program the crystal how long you want the treatment to go. If your friend Jack wants the half-hour treatment, you would simply either tell the crystal with your thoughts or voice to send Reiki to Jack for half an hour, or you could use your imagination to visualize Jack inside the crystal and then see a clock hand's turn to indicate half an hour. Remember, the crystal is infused with Divine consciousness, so you can speak to it verbally or with your mind. And, if speaking to it with your mind, you do not need to be an expert in visualization, or in telepathy with the crystal to get it to work as you wish. It will do so simply through your effort to make it happen. This is extremely important to note: the crystal is made up in part of Divine consciousness, a consciousness which probably knows what you are thinking before you even think it. So, you cannot do a visualization incorrectly, or make an error in programming the crystal with your thoughts or voice. It will know what to do. And it is simply your attention, your care, that is the essential ingredient to activate the crystal into sending the treatment.

Just think it or just say it, and the crystal will do the rest of the work. This is the fascinating and truly awakened power that is so amazing about Mikao Usui's Reiki Crystal of Awakening as a Reiki healing tool.

You can similarly send Reiki treatments backwards or forward in time to yourself or another using the same technique. The only variation is that you would need to be specific in your intention, thinking or vocally commanding the Reiki treatment to be for the past or the future, and be specific enough so that the treatment happens at the point in time you intend it to.

Practice this technique now on yourself, sending a Reiki treatment to yourself backwards in time.

Pick a moment in your life when you would like to have had some healing. Now, visualize yourself at that point in time, but seeing that point in time happening inside the Reiki crystal, almost like a movie. Or, if you are not a visual person, you can simply intend with your thoughts or gently whisper that the Reiki crystal send you a treatment backwards in time to a specific date or event. Be specific. Also, specify the amount of time you wish for the treatment to be. Then, lie back and relax once you have fully programmed the crystal with your intention. Often, even when sending a treatment backwards in time I will feel something happening in the present. Usually this may be a physical sensation, a lightening of an emotional charge about a past event, or other nuanced psychic data telling me that the energy is moving into the past and changing my experience of the past. Although this technique cannot actually change past events, it can change how you perceive and react to past events, even shifting your own memory to some degree.

The best way to understand this is simply to work with this technique over time and notice the subtle changes which occur when sending repeated Reiki treatments to the same, or similar, events from the past, events that may have been painful or harmful to you when they originally happened. Repeated treatments into the past can change how you feel about certain events. The emotional charge around traumatic events can be lessened, and in most cases entirely released.

Sending Reiki into the future is also very useful. The technique is the same as sending into the past. The only difference is that it may be more difficult for those who work with visualization to create an image in their mind's eye of something that has not yet happened. But, intention is truly all that is necessary. So, as long as you intend the treatment arrive in the future at a certain place or time, it will. I often enjoy sending treatments forward in time to work issues or meetings that I might otherwise expect to be stressful. Without fail, sending Reiki in such situations always makes the outcome smoother, easier, and more in alignment with the highest good.

Make a practice of sending Reiki using Mikao Usui's Reiki Crystal of Awakening every day. This will give you the opportunity to practice, and also teach you more about what is possible with this amazing Reiki crystal. Eventually, the crystal itself will become your true teacher, as you learn to listen to it on an intuitive level, knowing that the crystal is imbued with Divine consciousness, that it can actually communicate with you and teach you more than this author can ever do.

If the idea of sending Reiki is intimidating or confusing, start with some of the suggested treatments below. Once you gain a deeper sense of experience with the crystal, working with it on a daily basis will most likely become second nature to you and eventually require little or no effort at all.

Suggested treatments:

1   Whenever possible practice sending treatments to consenting friends, relatives or even willing acquaintances.

2   Send Reiki treatments backwards in time to yourself to any traumatic injury, or psychologically difficult time in your past. Repeat sending treatments to the same time in the past over and over until those situations in the past feel entirely free from any emotional charge.

3   Send Reiki treatments forward in time to your day. Making this a regular practice can be very uplifting and allows daily events to generally flow easier.

4   Send Reiki to bless your food. Simply imagine the plate of

food inside the Reiki crystal for a few minutes before each meal. You can also do the same with any liquids you consume, such as blessing a glass of water.

5   Send Reiki to yourself backwards in time to the moment your soul was first created by the Divine. (This can be a very mystical experience.) Do this by simply asking the Reiki crystal, since visualizing such a profound event can be challenging.

6   Send Reiki to your pets if you have any. I try to use my intuition to ask an animal first if they wish to receive Reiki, since there are some times when an animal may not want it, though usually they will welcome it.

7   Send Reiki to houseplants, and trees. One nice way to work with this is to send Reiki to an important tree in your life, maybe one you climbed during childhood. For those who have a strong psychic sense, sending Reiki to an important tree from your past can feel almost like having a conversation with a long-lost friend.

8   Be creative, play and try something new each day with the Reiki crystal. Remember, as long as you are not violating the free will of others by sending unwanted treatments, there is no harm that can come from sending Reiki. Be playful! Reiki practitioners can often be far too serious. Be joyful and see Reiki as a form of playing with the Divine.

Chapter 8

Meditating with Your Reiki Crystal

Mikao Usui's Reiki Crystal of Awakening is both a powerful crystal of Reiki light, and also a nexus point where your consciousness and Divine consciousness merge. This merging point allows you to use the crystal for meditative purposes, to deepen your spiritual awareness, and most importantly to teach you all that Mikao Usui's Reiki Crystal of Awakening is capable of doing.

You can use the Reiki crystal for meditative purposes simply by bringing your consciousness into the crystal through focusing your attention upon it. Simply focusing your attention upon the crystal automatically activates a level of communication between you and the crystal; a level of communication that not only allows you to give input to focus Reiki treatments on certain areas of the body, but also a level of communication which allows the crystal to interact with your own consciousness. This two-way communication is in itself one of the greatest benefits of this new form of Reiki. Although the symbols used in traditional Reiki are powerful and quite useful, they are in themselves not conscious. They are energetic devices, capable of bringing forth great healing, but they cannot offer wisdom or spiritual insights. But because Mikao Usui's Reiki Crystal of Awakening is imbued with Divine consciousness, it is capable of offering healing advice, wisdom and spiritual insight. Once you become fully in relationship with this crystal, it will be the only Reiki teacher you need.

You have already begun creating a relationship with this crystal through the work of the previous chapters. But so far that work has been primarily about using the crystal to perform Reiki treatments, to send Reiki either distantly or to bring greater focus for the Reiki treatments you have done in person. As noble as these functions are, they do not compare with what you will be able to explore with the crystal in this and future chapters.

Let's begin this deepening process with a simple meditation. Bring your awareness on to Mikao Usui's Reiki Crystal of Awakening, located a few inches in front of the center of your chest. Again, some of you may actually see the crystal as about the size of a golf ball, filled with a brilliant white light. Now, focus your intention on the crystal so that it brings you into a meditation. Or, if you are one who does not see the Reiki crystal you can ask the crystal, either with your mind or your voice, to bring you into a meditation. The crystal will react to the request, by bringing your consciousness into the crystal and merging it with the Divine consciousness already imbued into the crystal. Usually, this will result in a sense of calm and peace overcoming all else. You may have insights about your own life while in this deep peaceful state of consciousness. Let your consciousness rest there for several minutes. Take as long as you like. This place of consciousness is precious, loving, and eternally compassionate. Yet this is not the same as receiving a Reiki treatment. There is no Reiki energy flowing to you from the crystal at this point, but more that the crystal is literally sharing its own consciousness with yours.

Once you have tried the simple meditation technique above, you can then explore other meditative options with the crystal. Try working with the crystal now to deepen your own experience and knowledge of Reiki. The crystal can offer you insights on what you need to work on to deepen your Reiki practice. It can also offer suggestions for new Reiki techniques and creative ways of using existing techniques. Again, the crystal can do this because it is organized by Divine mind, and is imbued with Divine consciousness.

Bring your focus again on the Reiki crystal with this new intention that it offer you a meditation for deepening your own

Reiki practice. Again, all you need to do is focus your awareness on the crystal while mentally holding the above intention. Or, simply ask it to offer you a meditation to deepen your Reiki practice, asking with your mind or your voice. Make sure you allow for there to be enough time to fully engage and absorb the meditative experience. You may want to keep a journal nearby to write down and record the information you receive.

Another suggested way to use the crystal to deepen your Reiki practice is to ask the crystal to deepen your awareness of Mikao Usui's Five Principles of Reiki. The five principles are less about how to use Reiki energy, and are more a code of how a Reiki initiate should live and be in the world. In my own Reiki training, there was very little emphasis on these five principles such that for many years I all but ignored them. It was not until my own Reiki path deepened dramatically that I began to fully understand their importance to the overall system of Reiki, which is much more than just an energy healing system, but is a path to spiritual awakening.

Mikao Usui's Five Principles of Reiki are:

Just for today, I will not anger.
Just for today, I will not worry.
Just for today, I will show gratitude to every living thing.
Just for today, I will make my living honestly.
Just for today, I will be kind to every living thing.

Try meditating with the Reiki crystal to gain a deeper understanding of each principle, one at a time. In my own work with this, the Reiki crystal has helped me have an appreciation for these principles in ways that are much deeper than my intellect alone could discover. For example, I did not subscribe to these principles for many years because my own relationship with my parents was so dysfunctional that I did not know how not to be angry with them. Therefore, I dismissed the principle about not being angry and so did not focus on the five principles as a body of spiritual teaching. Yet in working with Mikao Usui's Reiki Crystal of Awakening, and the Forgiveness Reiki symbols from my book *Reiki for Spiritual Healing*, I was able to see simple ways in which transforming my anger towards my parents into positive actions for my own healing and searching for positive values for my own path was necessary for my own spiritual growth. That does not mean I have to be in or maintain a dysfunctional relationship. But, I have been able to move beyond my anger and transform it by making use of Reiki as a spiritual healing energy. So, using the Reiki crystal in this form of meditation allowed me to see the whole picture, and have a deeper understanding of this Reiki principle and its impact on my life.

Similar insights may come to you about any of these five principles, as long as you meditate on each one, using the Reiki crystal to deepen your understanding of each.

Chapter 9

Reiki on the Internet and in Daily Life

One of the reasons I offer this book is to see Reiki become much more a part of people's daily life experience. Reiki as a healing system for the most part is fairly complete using the traditional symbols and hand position sequences taught by thousands of Reiki Masters around the world. Although there are some very wonderful healing options that can be added using Reiki Higher Self techniques from my book *Reiki for Spiritual Healing*, and by using the techniques made available with Mikao Usui's Reiki Crystal of Awakening, for the most part the Reiki system as it has been taught for generations in itself is very complete for the purposes of a one on one practitioner/client healing relationship, or for self treatments.

However, since being initiated into Reiki twenty years ago it has amazed me that there are so many possibilities to bring Reiki into daily life that are often not explored in traditional Reiki trainings. Maybe that has been part of the reason I have been called to explore other possible Reiki functions, because I feel this wonderful powerful healing light should not be restricted to just a one on one healing session or a self treatment. I feel it is meant for daily human experiences, and is a Divine light that can raise the vibration of almost every human interaction. In my book *The Reiki Magic Guide to Self-Attunement* I even relate in detail some of my experiments with Reiki attunements of water and how that could be used in agriculture to stimulate healthier and more vibrant crops (these small experiments indicate it would actually be quite beneficial). My curiosity has always been in how to make Reiki not only more functional as a healing system, but also how to bring it into daily life and have this Divine light be part of most of our human experiences.

Similar to the way I have worked with attuning water to Reiki, and have found results being very positive, I have often felt drawn to attune inanimate objects to Reiki to improve their functioning. These experiments have included stones, radios, CD players and more. And always my experience has been that you can literally attune anything to Reiki. It does not have to be human, animal or even in accordance with the scientific definition of a living being. Yet, only recently have I begun to experiment with the intersection of attuning something that is inanimate and yet which interacts with billions of people across the planet daily: the Internet.

The concept of attuning the Internet to Reiki probably seems quite grandiose. And if it seemed like a secret I should keep to myself then I probably would, just to spare myself the ridicule of making such a claim. Yet this attunement was not something I felt like doing on a whim, but was something I was shown to do when almost on the cusp of falling asleep. It is in those times that I usually am taught the most radical energy healing techniques by my guides. Also, the techniques which will follow in this chapter reveal ways to make Reiki readily available to anyone with a computer.

Late in April of 2012, I was about to go to sleep and was shown on an energetic level the deep level of consciousness that exists in computers; that computers are an extension of the human mental body on a massive scale. I was also told by my guides in that moment that I should attune the World Wide Web of the Internet to Reiki. Since there is no one rightful owner of the Internet, and it is in the public domain, I asked the angels and devas of both Reiki and the Internet if this was for the highest good of all and was told that it was. So, in that moment I worked with these same angels and devas, and my higher self and all my Reiki guides to empower the Internet to Mikao Usui's Reiki Crystal of Awakening. Later the next day I sent a tweet that the World Wide Web was now attuned to Reiki.

What this means is that the Divine consciousness that exists within Mikao Usui's Reiki Crystal of Awakening, that same consciousness and energetic healing ability, can now be accessed through the Internet. There is no website to go to, no Facebook page or Twitter account to use or follow. It is the Internet itself.

The way anyone can access this is simply by being online on their laptop, mobile phone or any other device that connects to the Internet. Once online, you simply type into the body of an e-mail, or tweet, or Facebook update the exact details of the Reiki treatment you are requesting the Internet to send. The best way to experiment with this concept, which is certainly at the edge of what most people may be willing to believe, is to go online and type into a Google search engine the following phrase: *The Internet is sending me Reiki as I look at this page.* Then, without actually performing a Google search simply sit in front of your computer and allow the Internet to send you Reiki. Again, if you are someone who does not sense energy healing it will be very unlikely that this concept will make much sense, as I admit it is at the edge of what one might find believable. Yet if you are one who is energy sensitive my experience is that you will feel Reiki begin to flow to you once you have typed in the phrase into the search bar.

How this works is that once it was empowered to Mikao Usui's Reiki Crystal of Awakening the Internet's own consciousness, however mechanical or evolved it may be, also merged to some degree with the Divine consciousness that exists in the Reiki crystal. So, when you type into an e-mail, or Facebook update, or any place on the Internet any kind of command or request that the Internet send Reiki, that request is activated within Mikao Usui's Reiki Crystal of Awakening. However, instead of projecting that thought into your own Reiki crystal you are projecting it into the Reiki crystal that now exists within the Internet itself. And, as you have experienced so far in this book, it is when your own thoughts are projected into the

Reiki crystal that the healing is activated.

Another way to look at this issue is that the Internet is a physical representation of the group mind of all who use it. So, by attuning the Internet, the physical representation of that group mind, it isn't that every computer or every person hooked in to the Internet is now a Reiki practitioner. But that this shared wisdom, this collective of ideas and thoughts, is now imbued with Divine consciousness and an energetic Reiki crystal that will allow anyone who wishes to access Reiki to be able to do so through the Internet.

Again, my Reiki theories are always backed up by experiment. So, if you are one who senses energy healing, then go to your computer now and try the above experiment on your own. If you are one who does not experience any sensation from energy healing, then gather those friends or acquaintances you know who do feel energy healing, and ask them to perform the same experiment.

When performing the experiment it is important to write that the *Internet* is sending the treatment. If you make the mistake of writing the statement without specifically indicating that the Internet is sending the treatment, the experiment will not work. Also, make sure you are typing into some system directly connected and online at the moment you are writing it. In other words, typing the phrase into a word document will not have any impact, since that is an internal software of your computer, not a component of the Internet. In order for the experiment to work, the typed phrase must be directly input into an Internet search engine, e-mail account, or some form of social media account that is active and online.

Once you have tried the experiment and understand that it does work, you can then use this form of Reiki as a supplement to bring Reiki into daily life. I would never use this technique for a professional Reiki healing. But I would use it for things like helping release stress during a difficult day at work, by simply typing into the body of an e-mail to myself that the Internet is sending Reiki to me in my office for ten minutes. I use this kind of technique during a day when I will not have time to send Reiki to myself, but when I do have a spare few seconds to type out an e-mail. Try it and see for yourself the impact it can have on reducing stress in the workplace.

Another way to use this technique is to e-mail short mini Reiki treatments to friends and family. This is not intended to diminish the value or sacredness of a deep one on one Reiki healing. But instead, it is intended to awaken both the one receiving the treatment as well as the one sending the e-mail that Reiki is available to us always, and that the Divine is present with us even during the most mundane aspects of our daily lives.

Play with this idea and see what your own results may be. When I first shared this concept with one of my friends and disclosed to her how it worked, for a few minutes it was very tempting to think of how this could be turned into a Reiki app, a Reiki video game and other such options that would have been more about me and others making money than about any sense of expanding the possibilities of Reiki to a wider circle. But my sense is that this is information that is meant to be shared freely, and not something which could end up as a trade secret should I have opted to take this to an ambitious software developer instead of a reputable book publisher.

Play with the following Internet Reiki options:

1   Write into an e-mail that the Internet will send a Reiki energetic clearing to your home or office.
2   Send an e-mail Reiki mini treatment to a friend (as long as you have their permission to do so).
3   Create a Reiki group on social media that promotes and uses these Reiki Internet techniques to send Reiki to larger world issues. Imagine, a million people with a Facebook status update where they are sending Reiki to

world peace... how that might impact the consciousness of our world at large.

The possibilities are endless. The only limit, as long as you are respecting free will, is your own imagination.

Chapter 10

The Reiki Sphere of Divine Grace

Mikao Usui's Reiki Crystal of Awakening is continuously evolving, which makes it both a wonderful spiritual tool and yet also challenging to describe in full. In essence, no one will ever be able to capture all the techniques or possibilities of this crystal into one book. Even as I write this book now, the information about the crystal is changing so rapidly that at times I feel I am going to have to delete chapters I have just written, because new information that will make them obsolete is arising at the same time I am writing. One technique, however, that I cannot imagine becoming obsolete is a technique I discovered just recently while in the midst of experimenting with the Reiki crystal. This technique is one I call the Reiki Sphere of Divine Grace.

The Reiki Sphere of Divine Grace is literally a sphere of Reiki light generated by the Reiki crystal. This sphere envelopes a person entirely, and feels as close as one can imagine to being held by the Divine. It is a blissful, nurturing healing session all by itself, but can also be integrated with other Reiki techniques. Try experiencing this now by simply asking Mikao Usui's Reiki Crystal of Awakening to surround you with the Reiki Sphere of Divine Grace. You can make this request either audibly, or simply with your thoughts, as long as the request is specifically made to the Reiki crystal.

Once the request is given, the Reiki crystal will begin creating a sphere of Reiki light totally surrounding you. The sphere will usually be a few feet wider and taller than you are. Also, it usually takes a few seconds to be generated; so it does not appear instantly, but instead grows out of the Reiki crystal until you are surrounded by it.

Once you are surrounded by it, simply let go, knowing there

is nowhere to be, nothing to do, nothing to achieve. You are simply immersed in a sphere of Reiki light that is a full embodiment of Divine Grace. Be with it! Enjoy it! And allow it to rid you of stress, worry and any type of fear. The beauty of the Reiki Sphere of Divine Grace is that lower vibrations, such as fear and worry, simply cannot exist within the sphere, and simply melt away.

Use the Reiki sphere on yourself before going to bed, or at a time when you can deeply relax without needing to have anything else on your agenda for hours. It is truly the most beautiful form of Reiki energy I have ever experienced, and is so easy to experience: all you have to do is ask the Reiki crystal, and you shall receive.

Chapter 11

Teaching Reiki to Others

Mikao Usui's Reiki Crystal of Awakening carries within it the ability to empower others to Reiki. It can do this in several ways. It can either be used to attune one to Reiki levels as taught in the traditional system of Reiki, as first, second or third degree Reiki attunements. Or it can create a replica of itself within another person, manifesting a Reiki crystal a few inches in front of the center of another person's chest, and thus giving that person access to all the possibilities of Mikao Usui's Reiki Crystal of Awakening. My own sense is that the latter is preferred, and that Reiki as a system is evolving to a place where it will eventually be taught primarily as a one degree system, with no hierarchy at all.

To use the Reiki crystal for empowering another to Mikao Usui's Reiki Crystal of Awakening, simply ask the crystal to perform the empowerment and it will do so. It is incredibly easy, fast, and user friendly. There are no complex symbols to memorize, no sequences of breaths and hand motions to know. Again, because this form of Reiki is truly an embodiment of Divine grace, all you need to do as the Reiki teacher is ask for the empowerment to happen and it will. What happens during the empowerment is the Reiki crystal literally manifests a replica of itself within the other person's energy field. Know that although I refer to it as a replica, it is just as powerful and just as real as the original version of Mikao Usui's Reiki Crystal of Awakening, which I was blessed to receive several years ago. In fact, my belief is that there is actually only one Reiki crystal, and that the miracle of Reiki is that that one crystal exists in many places simultaneously, existing in each of us who are willing to accept this form of Divine grace. But, for the sake of working within the four-dimensional universe as we humans experience it, I tend to think of the crystal as creating a replica of itself, which makes it easier for my mind to comprehend.

The attunement process involves you first making the request to the crystal to attune another to Mikao Usui's Reiki Crystal of Awakening. Once the crystal receives the request, it begins sending an extension of itself, almost like a solar flare, into the energy field of the person who is being initiated. The initiate's energy system is then downloaded with the energetic program of Divine light that creates the crystal. While the crystal is being created with this program of Divine light, it is important to invite the initiate to perform a very simple function or two using the crystal.

You will want to describe the crystal to them first, telling them it is a ball of Reiki light about the size of a golf ball, existing a few inches in front of the center of their chest. Let them know that the ball of light is literally a crystal of Divine light, which can be programmed collaboratively with their consciousness and the consciousness of the Divine. Ask them to perform a very simple task, such as imagining their mind or brain inside the crystal and then intending the crystal to bathe their mind with Reiki light. Any request will do, as the purpose is to simply activate the crystal and have the person begin using it while it is still being formed. In essence, you are wanting the person to imprint their own thoughts upon the crystal and begin forming a relationship with it.

After you have asked the person to perform a simple function or two, you will likely have completed the empowerment. You will know the empowerment is complete when energy is no longer flowing from the Reiki crystal in front of your chest out to the person you are empowering.

Once the person is empowered, take them through some of the exercises mentioned in Chapters Three, Four and Five of this book. Ideally, you would want to make this book available to the student, since it is the only text written that reveals these Reiki crystal techniques. But, should a book not be available, at least teach the person how to perform a basic self treatment as well as a treatment on another person. From there, they will at least gain a substantial benefit from the empowerment, and hopefully then have a steady enough understanding of the Reiki crystal to begin to trust it as their own teacher. Which is what all who read this book should aspire to: making Mikao Usui's Reiki Crystal of Awakening your teacher for learning all that it can offer.

Should you decide to offer workshops in the techniques shown in this book, that is welcomed as long as you mention the source of this work and this book as the primary text. Please know, as mentioned in the initial portion of this chapter, that the Reiki crystal can also empower, initiate and attune individuals to the traditional levels of Reiki as well. And although I do not see that as its primary purpose, it can be a benefit for those who are trained and qualified as teachers of traditional Reiki should they want to use this method as an easier form of attunement process.

Should you wish to use the crystal to perform a Reiki attunement of one of the traditional Reiki levels, simply imagine the person you are wishing to attune to Reiki inside of the Reiki crystal. Then, either out loud or with your mind, ask the Reiki crystal to initiate or attune the person to whichever specified level of Reiki you wish to confer upon the individual. You may then feel the Reiki symbols moving inside the crystal as the attunement process takes place. Using the Reiki crystal to pass traditional Reiki attunements is intended to be used more as a technique of convenience among established Reiki Masters, one that is far less time consuming than techniques from the past, but which can offer the same level of result. If you have not been trained as a traditional Reiki Master, and have no knowledge of the Reiki symbols or their use, then I would not recommend engaging the Reiki crystal in this manner. It is simply offered here as a tool of convenience for those who are trained in traditional Reiki symbols and their use.

Chapter 12

Reiki for Sexual Healing

Reiki is powerful, loving and can be profoundly useful in healing sexual trauma. And most of us have some form of sexual trauma, even if just the social restrictions placed upon us because of our gender. Though for many of us, that sexual trauma has been more severe in situations of rape, incest and childhood sexual abuse. For years I have avoided teaching some Reiki techniques I knew were real and powerful, simply because of the social and cultural stigma involved around sex, as well as the unfortunate stories about some who abuse their power even within the community of Reiki. I did not want to give tools to those who might misuse them to sexually exploit others. And yet as a survivor of sexual abuse, I have fully welcomed the healing I have received from Reiki with regards to my sexuality. The beauty of Mikao Usui's Reiki Crystal of Awakening is that it has allowed me to offer techniques that I feel are entirely safe and respectful, and yet which can be done with deep reverence. These techniques can happen simply between you and yourself, as a way to heal your own body of old sexual trauma; or they can happen between you and a lover, as a way to deepen the sacred sexual bond between you both.

The first Reiki technique for sexual healing is to cleanse the sexual organs of all negative memories or energies. This can be done through a simple request to the Reiki crystal. Simply ask with your mind, or ask audibly, that the Reiki crystal cleanse your sexual organs of all unwanted memories and all negative energies. Remember, the crystal is a culmination of all Reiki intelligence, all Reiki techniques, and is imbued with Divine consciousness. So, you don't need to micromanage it, but simply give it the instructions of the end goal, which in this case is to cleanse the sexual organs of all unwanted memories and all negative energies. The crystal may send Reiki through time into your pelvic area, or it may run a deep treatment on your sexual organs, which runs along an entire time line of negative experiences. Or it may run deep into the cellular memory of your penis or vagina to release old emotional scars held in those parts of the body, or it may send Reiki backwards in time to a particular traumatic event in the past. But most likely the Reiki crystal will do all of the above, simultaneously, and more. Again, that is the beauty of this multidimensional, conscious form of Reiki: that it can do many things at once.

Try asking the Reiki crystal to perform this cleansing on a regular basis; and if you have major trauma held in your sexual organs, notice how quickly that trauma may begin to dissolve and release with repeated treatments. Again, there is no need to micromanage the crystal, which has Divine consciousness within it and will know the best techniques to use for the deepest and most effective healing possible. In addition, repeating this process on a regular basis will also release any negative social programming about your sexuality that may be held energetically in those same areas. So, even if you do not have any past sexual trauma, using this technique can still have the benefit of releasing negative programming from teachers, parents, or society in general. Often we take in insults towards our gender and internalize them energetically in the sexual organs. Simple taunts from childhood about being a boy or a girl can be held energetically in or near the genitals, and carried with us through our entire life. Or, similarly, social expectations about having to perform as a male, or about having to suppress your sexuality as a female, are also often held in these areas. Using this technique can help release those energetic chains, and allow us to become truly sexually liberated and free.

A second technique I recommend, with respect to using Reiki to heal sexual trauma, is to ask the Reiki crystal to clear any energetic cords or psychological bonds between yourself and anyone who sexually mistreated you. These cords exist in any instance where there has been sexual contact, even casual sexual encounters. Therefore, it is an important area to address with respect to sexual healing. In fact, in my own healing journey it was when I began clearing the energetic cords between myself and my childhood abusers that I began to actually move beyond my past and feel free from it. As effective as psychological treatment can be in overcoming sexual trauma, it is rare that these cords will be dealt with or even recognized through traditional therapy. Usually, it takes a shaman or adept energy healer to even recognize the need for this level of healing. But this form of healing does need to happen, because until the cords are cleared there is still an energetic connection between an abuse survivor and the abuser. Using the Reiki crystal to clear these cords is an important step forward in the healing process. Also, it is important to note that this technique does not have to be reserved for issues of profound abuse such as rape or incest. It can also be used to clear away energetic attachments to any former partner who was not nurturing enough, or who reinforced negative patterns, or someone who you may simply regret to have shared yourself with. The Reiki crystal can work to clear any of these.

The way this treatment works is you can either visualize yourself and the other person inside the Reiki crystal, a few inches in front of the center of your chest, intending that the Reiki crystal clear out any energy cords between the two of you. Or, a much simpler way would be to simply ask the crystal audibly to clear any energy cords between you and the other person.

The way the treatment works is that the Reiki crystal is illuminating all energetic attachments and energetic cords between you and the other person, and then transforming these energetic attachments and cords into pure light. You may feel old memories arise, or repressed emotions come to the surface during this process. Be patient, and know that even if something uncomfortable comes to the surface it will be transformed by the Reiki crystal.

Allow the treatment to run its course. Usually, it will take only a few minutes. In some cases you may need to repeat the treatment more than once before the situation is fully cleared. You will know it is fully cleared when there is no longer any emotional charge if thinking about the person in question. Depending on the nature and depth of what needs to be released, it may be something you can release with a few short treatments, or something that requires more ongoing repeated treatments. Be patient if you are clearing a situation that happened over the course of months or years, or if there was extreme violence involved. Reiki is capable of healing even the deepest and most disturbing trauma, but please give yourself and the Reiki crystal the time and space to make these changes occur. Although I have personally experienced small energetic miracles when doing this kind of work, I have found it is best not to expect them. Be patient enough to know that the process itself is what heals, and being *dedicated* to an ongoing healing process is in itself perhaps the most important aspect of the healing, knowing that you are truly committed to heal no matter how much time and effort is required.

Chapter 13

Reiki at Work

I have been a proponent for many years that Reiki is not just a tool for individual sessions, but that it is also a means by which we can bring Divine light into every aspect of our being. One such way to do that is to bring Reiki into your work environment. In my role at Omega Institute, I have often been complimented on how well I handle my job. Often, those who had previously been in the same role would reach psychological burnout within months, or become bitter at the energetic onslaught of having two hundred staff members always wanting their attention. But I have been in the role for over a decade, and have found that a great ingredient for my success has been my ability to use Reiki in the workplace. This does not mean I have been sending Reiki treatments to people that I work with, which I certainly would not do without their consent. But it does mean that there are Reiki techniques for shifting the energy of a situation, an important meeting, even changing the ambience of a room, which can be important tools for those in high stress work situations.

Now that you have access to Mikao Usui's Reiki Crystal of Awakening, you can literally ask it for direct assistance and input on just about any matter at work. If a difficult issue arises, simply allow your consciousness to sink into the Reiki crystal for a meditation, or if it is easier just ask the crystal out loud that it pull your consciousness into a Reiki meditation on the issue at hand. Try this process now just to experiment with it. First, think about an issue you have at work. Then once you have fully focused on that issue, ask Mikao Usui's Reiki Crystal of Awakening to take you into a Reiki meditation to help you find peace with the issue at hand.

When I try this process myself I usually feel a sense of

pressure in the area of my head. It feels like a strong Reiki presence, but is not the same as receiving a flow of Reiki energy. Remember, the Reiki crystal is imbued with Divine consciousness. So this process is much deeper than if it were simply Reiki energy bathing your mind to allow you to come to your own resolution. In this instance the Reiki crystal is communicating with you. It is doing so by forming a Reiki hologram of your own brain, infused with the wisdom the crystal has to offer, then merging that Reiki hologram in with your own brain so that the information is transferred directly to you. Your ability to fully recognize the information is still subject to your own mental filters, and therefore cannot be considered fail proof or accurate one hundred percent of the time. This is because the information from the Reiki crystal still has to be interpreted by your own mind, which is also influenced by your subconscious mind. The information itself will always be highly accurate and beneficial, but since it must be *interpreted* through your own mental filters beware if you think you are hearing the crystal telling you to suddenly quit your job, play the lotto, or do anything rash or extravagant. In fact, the crystal will never really tell you what to do at all; it will only present images and pictures of various possibilities. Still, it can be a fabulous tool for presenting options you may not have considered.

When using the Reiki crystal in this way you may want to have a journal with you and write down notes. Please know the crystal does not make predictions of the future, nor does it serve as a resident psychic existing a few inches in front of you. What it does, quite simply, is bring into your awareness possible ways of approaching a problem. That is all. It is always your responsibility in the end to decide what to do with the information.

Another way you can use the Reiki crystal in the workplace is to ask the Reiki crystal to optimize the energetic flow in your work environment. To do this, simply imagine your work environment inside of the Reiki crystal and then intend the crystal work to optimize the energetic flow. Or, you can use the voice-activated approach of simply asking out loud that the crystal optimize the energetic flow of your work environment. Either approach will do. Once you have made the request, either out loud or through visualization with the Reiki crystal, then just relax and allow the crystal to do its work. Usually a treatment will run for a matter of minutes. Treatments should be repeated either daily, or as needed.

Reiki optimization of the workplace can take many forms. Generally, it will make things flow smoother. Communication between coworkers will be easier. Tasks may come into alignment better and with a better sense of flow. I think of it as hitting the reset button. When the energy of an office or workplace has become frantic, it is easier for people to make mistakes and fall out of their own natural rhythm. Using the Reiki crystal to optimize the energetic flow helps reset the energy so that things flow naturally, more gets done and yet people seem more relaxed and more friendly in the process.

If you have a serious issue in the workplace, you can also use the Reiki crystal to assist with healing or resolving that issue. To do this, simply imagine the issue inside of the Reiki crystal, or use the voice-activated technique and simply ask the Reiki crystal to work on the issue. The Reiki crystal will then begin sending Reiki to the issue. This is not the same as sending Reiki to each individual person involved with the issue, but is more like praying or asking for Divine grace in the form of Reiki to become present in a situation. The presence of this Divine grace will usually cause people to act with more civility, and reorganize the energetic patterns present in the issue so that they bend more towards the highest good.

This process is not a cure-all panacea, however. If you have an abusive coworker, it may be that the Reiki crystal will show you a way to a new job with a better work environment. Or, it may lead the coworker to be let go by the management so they have to deal with the consequences of their own abusive behavior. It is often a mistake to think Reiki is always going to smooth things out and make life easy. If a situation that has been avoided requires an uncomfortable resolution, Reiki will call forth that uncomfortable resolution, as long as it is for the highest good.

Use the Reiki crystal to send Reiki to optimize the flow of the workplace, help resolve work issues, and meditate on the possibilities. A good practice is to use the Reiki crystal at least once per day at work, even if it is just to send Reiki to your workday. Remember, making this an ongoing practice will change your life for the better.

Chapter 14

Reiki and Food

A wonderful way to use Mikao Usui's Reiki Crystal of Awakening is to clear the energy of everything you eat and drink of any negative vibrations, as well as optimize the food and drink for your own digestion. We are what we eat, and by clearing the energy of food, and energetically aligning it with our own bodies, we are taking better care of ourselves.

The simple way to clear your food before each meal is to imagine the plate in front of you as inside the Reiki crystal, then intend that the crystal clear the food. Or use the voice-activated Reiki technique and simply ask the Reiki crystal to clear the food. Once the crystal begins its work, it normally will take only a few seconds to complete the task. What is happening when the crystal does this is that any negative thoughts or vibrations that may have merged into the food, from the farmhand all the way to the cook, are released. If you have ever eaten a meal prepared by an angry family member, you will know what it is like to eat food that carries a negative vibration within it. Since we cannot track our food from the farm all the way through to the time it is prepared, making use of this technique is a good practice to keep your body and energy field clear from unwanted negative vibrations.

Energetically clearing food is something that has been a common Reiki practice for generations. It is often taught in traditional Reiki training. However, the Reiki crystal can also be a technique for optimizing the food for your body. This technique can be done either simultaneously or separately from the food clearing technique. To activate this, simply use the visualization or voice-activated Reiki request; then the Reiki crystal will begin altering the vibrations in the food so that they are the best energetic match for your body. Please know this technique cannot change a food allergy, nor can it add vitamins that do not exist in certain foods. But it can radically alter the energetic signature of any kind of food. And just as homeopathic medicine is based on the concept of energy signatures having a profound effect on the human body, so too can you alter and optimize the energy signature of everything you eat so that it becomes the optimal food for your body.

This is different than simply releasing a negative thought or negative vibration from food. When we are releasing a negative thought or vibration from food we are taking out something that is foreign to the overall vibration of the food itself. When we are changing the vibration of the food, the energy of the food itself is being changed.

A perfect example of this is that for many years at Omega Institute I would play a game with another energy healer friend of mine. The two of us would use Reiki or other energy techniques to add to or change the energetic vibration in a glass of water; then ask the other to guess what the change was. Often, we were fairly accurate in being able to guess what kind of energy healing had been added to the water, and how the energetic signature of the glass of water had been altered. Over the years I came to realize that this game actually had a great potential to shift and alter the energetic vibration of food to be optimal for the person consuming it. The Reiki crystal, as an advanced energy healing tool, has taken this a step even further. Previously, I had to consciously direct the energetic signature changes and hope that they would be optimal for myself, or the friend who was drinking the glass of water. But now, since the Reiki crystal is imbued with Divine consciousness, it can make these changes on its own for the highest good. All you have to do is make the request, and the Reiki crystal will do the rest.

It is natural to be skeptical of these kinds of unscientific claims. So, try your own experiment. Use the Reiki crystal at every meal for twenty-one days to clear the food of each meal, and also to optimize the vibration of your food for each meal. Then, keep a journal on how you feel physically. Note the days when you are lethargic, and the days when you feel energized. It may not seem that noticeable in the beginning, but track it regardless, taking a daily inventory of how you feel, and how your body is reacting to this process. Then, at the end of the twenty-one days stop using the Reiki crystal in this manner, and just eat as you did before using these techniques. Yet continue journaling about how you feel, how your body feels. Go for one full week without clearing your food at all, and without using the Reiki crystal to optimize your food for consumption. Then, once you have gone for a full week without using the Reiki crystal to clear your food, decide and be the judge of whether or not it was effective during the twenty-one day period. My sense is the vast majority or people will find that the Reiki crystal technique for clearing and optimizing food vibrations is highly effective, and they will resume using it once they have tried this. The reason I ask you to try it this way is that sometimes we do not truly notice or appreciate something until we are without it. So, try using the Reiki crystal on your food for three weeks, then go one week without using it. I am certain you will be amazed at the difference.

Chapter 15

Reiki and Death

It may seem odd to include a chapter about death in a book that is about improving our day-to-day life. But I add this chapter to come full circle. Death is so deeply feared in the United States, much more so than in other parts of the world where death is not hidden, but accepted as part of the cycle of life. In my travels to Bali, where I once witnessed a human cremation ceremony that celebrated the passing of a person's spirit from this realm to the next, I then saw for the first time that not all cultures deny death or rage against it the way we do in this culture. For the Balinese, and some other cultures, death is a part of the larger cycle of life. I feel the same is true when it comes to Reiki.

One of the most beautiful things I often hear about when speaking to other Reiki Masters is how Reiki can be used to assist the dying to peacefully pass from this realm to the next. I first heard of this many years ago when I was only a second degree Reiki practitioner, and other Reiki practitioners in the town where I lived spoke about how they assisted energetically in the passing of a friend of theirs who was in the final stages of his struggle with HIV. I did not really comprehend this at first. And later, as my Reiki journey continued, I heard similar stories more and more about how Reiki did not always cure an illness, but sometimes actually helped move a person on from a place of suffering into the peaceful realm of death. Over the next few years I spent time sending Reiki to the dying, at a hospice in Portland, Oregon, and then also at a hospice I worked with in San Francisco. The past few years I have been sending Reiki regularly to people with HIV through the Cambodian AIDS Project, not with the false hope of curing anyone's illness but to assist them in moving beyond their suffering in this life and onwards into the light on the other side. It is not that I intend anyone to die during the treatments, but that I surrender to that sense of Divine grace which is present even in the process of death. Such treatments can work to alleviate suffering, and also in some cases help a person let go enough from their attachments to this life and onwards to continue their spiritual journey in the afterlife.

Death is something I fear, even as much as I want to embrace it and be at peace with it. Yet in my attempt to work through this fear I have sent layers and layers of Reiki treatments over the years to the point in time in the future when I pass away from this life. On days when I have nothing pressing on my agenda, I often will send a five- or ten-minute Reiki treatment forward in time to the point of my own death. Doing this may sound a bit morbid at first, but it actually is quite beautiful. It gives me a sense of my own mortality, but in a way that is still deeply connected with the Divine. It gives me the wisdom of knowing that when I do die, I will be washed in a wave of this healing spiritual light called Reiki during that process of dying. I know I will not feel alone, but will be filled with a sense of Divine grace when that time comes.

This does not mean I am in any way eager to die, but that Reiki has assisted me in accepting my own limits as a human being; the fact that I will one day no longer exist in a physical body. The work of sending Reiki forward in time to your own death may not be something you are right now ready to do, but I present it here simply as an option. It may be that your own way of coming to terms with death is simply to offer Reiki to those in need who are in the process of dying, be that a loved one in your own life or a stranger at a hospice or hospital. Or, it may be that you have no interest at all in even thinking about death, and so may want to dismiss this chapter all together. Yet I present this information here simply to acknowledge the presence of death, and bring it into the conversation about Reiki. For even before I began to explore alternate Reiki techniques, I often used traditional Reiki symbols to send Reiki forward in time to my own death, my own process of dying. And it is something I have never regretted. For it is in honoring death that we truly can live, and can know the gorgeous qualities of each moment.

If you feel ready, the following exercise is intended for those who are willing to use Reiki to face their own death directly, as well as bring healing forward in time to the process of their own dying. If this feels too strange, then there is no need to pressure yourself: simply stop reading this chapter or go ahead and read and do the exercise later in your life when it feels appropriate. But for those who are ready, the following exercise can be a fascinating journey.

Start by bringing your consciousness into Mikao Usui's Reiki Crystal of Awakening and intend that the crystal begin sending a Reiki treatment forward in time to the moment of your own death. Allow this treatment to run for at least five or ten minutes. You may sense yourself forward in time, either just prior to death, during the process of death, or immediately after death. You may also experience all of these in consecutive stages. Simply allow yourself to witness, and know the intent of the Reiki treatment is not to prolong your life or keep Death at bay, but to bring acceptance and peace to your own consciousness during the process of dying.

Once you have sent a Reiki treatment to the moment of your own death, shift the focus slightly so that the focus of the treatment is to send Reiki to your spirit just after the moment of death, with the intention that this treatment assist you in coping with your own death. In some circles it is believed that ghosts are simply spirits who have refused to acknowledge or accept their own death. Sending this kind of treatment can assist you in the future to not be stuck in a place of limbo or where you cannot move forward on to the next plane of existence after death. You may even wish to visualize yourself moving into the light, as is commonly mentioned by those who have had near-death experiences.

Reiki treatments sent forward in time towards your own death and dying process can be very healing, if only to shift your perception of death away from the fear-based impression so often culturally ingrained in our psyches. Once you can face death, using the above Reiki techniques, you can then begin to have a deeper appreciation for your own life, and each precious moment that you are existing in a human body. So, oddly enough, the healing you send forward to the process of your own death actually has the effect of empowering you to live more fully in the present, to embrace your life and live it with passion and purpose. Also, there is the side benefit of knowing that at the moment when you do die, you have already set into motion a wave of Reiki, a healing wave of Divine grace that will wash over you when the time of your passing occurs.

Use this process at your own convenience. It is not something to rush into if it makes you uncomfortable. But know that if used consciously it can help alleviate some of the underlying tension we often carry in this culture about death; this false sense that somehow we can fight it off and live forever. In time, you will gain perspective on your life journey when using this process repeatedly and with focused intention. It may help unfold your life purpose, and bring you insights you may never have imagined.

Chapter 16

Reiki for World Peace

One of my dreams as a Reiki Master has always been that if enough people who are empowered with Reiki actually organized and used their common ability to send Reiki towards the focused goal of world peace, that this goal could be achieved. Many Reiki healers around the globe send Reiki to their communities and Reiki for world peace. I applaud those who do this work, and I offer the following treatment simply as a way to continue that work now using Mikao Usui's Reiki Crystal of Awakening.

The below treatment is one which you can activate at any time. Please know it is my own belief as well that for us to have peace between human beings, we must also end our own war upon the planet. Peace for humans will not exist until there is also peace for all beings we share this planet with. We cannot as a species be at war with the rainforest, and at war with the oceans and still expect to be at peace with each other. Also, we cannot expect peace where there is injustice. Therefore, this treatment is also designed to work on the issues of world peace being attained by creating a just and peaceful world.

Reiki for World Peace Treatment

Mikao Usui's Reiki Crystal of Awakening is sending Reiki to bring peace and justice to humanity in all relationships with other living beings.

To activate the Reiki world peace treatment in your own Reiki crystal, simply say out loud:

I would like to invite Mikao Usui's Reiki Crystal of Awakening to send the Reiki for World Peace treatment for the next [state how many] *minutes.*

Once the treatment is invoked, then simply notice the energy move out from your Reiki crystal. You may also experience sensations, thoughts, images about world peace as the Reiki energy flows. Repeat as often as you like, and whenever you wish to contribute to the energy of world peace.

Chapter 17

Reiki Treatment Menu

The following is a menu of 88 Reiki treatment exercises that are programmed into Mikao Usui's Reiki Crystal of Awakening. Each has its own purpose, and can be activated simply by requesting mentally or audibly that the Reiki crystal perform the specific healing exercise. Since the Reiki crystal is imbued with Divine intelligence, all you need to do is specify the number on the Reiki menu and the name of the person (or being) who is receiving the treatment. The Reiki crystal will automatically do the rest.

These exercises are also designed to deepen your awareness of all that is possible with Mikao Usui's Reiki Crystal of Awakening. Practicing all of these exercises is recommended, even the ones that may seem unnecessary or beyond the norm of traditional Reiki healing sessions. Practicing all of them will broaden your own wisdom of how this crystal can be used for healing, spiritual growth, and daily living. And, since Reiki is guided by Divine intelligence, it can do no harm to try even the ones that seem unrelated to your present need or life situation.

It is important to note as well that there is a Reiki energetic signature for everything in existence. So, in some of the later treatments you will experience the Reiki of certain stones, crystals, herbs and sacred objects. Know that in all these instances the primary energy is still Reiki, just that it is being run through the prism of something already manifested in this world of form. That does not detract from the power of the Reiki energy, but simply focuses the energy for a more specific purpose. In the end the Divine consciousness in the Reiki crystal is in charge of the healing. So trust in the process, and know you are being held in an energetic form of Divine grace that is capable of expressing itself in myriad forms and manifestations.

To activate any of the below Reiki menu options, simply tell the Reiki crystal the number of the Reiki treatment you wish to receive, like ordering off a menu at a restaurant. You can use the following phrase to activate a treatment for yourself:

> *I would like Mikao Usui's Reiki Crystal of Awakening to send me Reiki Treatment number* [fill in the number].

Or, you can use the Reiki treatment menu for sending a treatment to someone else:

> *I would like Mikao Usui's Reiki Crystal of Awakening to send* [name of person] *Reiki Treatment number* [fill in the number].

It is that simple! Playing with these options gives you a deeper sense of the many possibilities with your Reiki crystal. And, know that in the end there are many more options than are on this Reiki menu. This menu of 88 choices is just the beginning.

Reiki Treatment #1: Mikao Usui's Reiki Crystal of Awakening is sending Reiki to your karmic body, using all Reiki lights designed to heal and release karmic debris and accelerate karmic cleansing. This treatment will last approximately thirty minutes, and will end with Mikao Usui's Reiki Crystal of Awakening performing integration Reiki for the last seven minutes of the healing.

Reiki Treatment #2: Mikao Usui's Reiki Crystal of Awakening is sending Reiki to your emotional body, using all Reiki lights designed to heal and release emotional issues. This treatment will last approximately thirty minutes and will end with Mikao Usui's Reiki Crystal of Awakening performing integration Reiki for the last seven minutes of the healing.

Reiki Treatment #3: Mikao Usui's Reiki Crystal of Awakening is sending Reiki to your mental body, using all Reiki lights designed to heal and release issues held in the mental body. This treatment will last approximately thirty minutes and will end with Mikao Usui's Reiki Crystal of Awakening performing integration Reiki for the last seven minutes of the healing.

Reiki Treatment #4: Mikao Usui's Reiki Crystal of Awakening is sending Reiki to all the meridians of your body, clearing all energetic obstacles from the meridians. This treatment will last approximately thirty minutes and will end with Mikao Usui's Reiki Crystal of Awakening performing integration Reiki for the last seven minutes of the healing.

Reiki Treatment #5: Mikao Usui's Reiki Crystal of Awakening is sending Reiki to clear all your chakras of all psychic or energetic debris. This treatment will last approximately twenty minutes and will end with Mikao Usui's Reiki Crystal of Awakening performing integration Reiki for the last five minutes of the healing.

Reiki Treatment #6: Mikao Usui's Reiki Crystal of Awakening is sending Reiki to your skeletal system for ten minutes, followed by sending Reiki to your muscles for ten minutes, followed by sending Reiki to your circulatory system for ten minutes, followed by sending Reiki to your respiratory system for ten minutes, followed by sending Reiki to your nervous system for ten minutes. And, this treatment will end with Mikao Usui's Reiki Crystal of Awakening performing integration Reiki for the last ten minutes of the healing.

Reiki Treatment #7: Mikao Usui's Reiki Crystal of Awakening is sending a Reiki energy clearing between [name of person] and [name of other person], to release all unwanted memories, negative energy and psychic attachments, from this life or any other lifetime. This treatment will run for forty minutes and will end with Mikao Usui's Reiki Crystal of Awakening performing integration Reiki for the last ten minutes of the healing.

Please note that when clearing the energy between two individuals it is only necessary to have the consent of one of them. Since energy is not being sent directly to either party, it is not in violation of anyone's personal space or physical being if only one of them consents.

Reiki Treatment #8: Mikao Usui's Reiki Crystal of Awakening is sending you a Reiki treatment for mending a broken heart, to release all wounds of the heart from this lifetime and transform them into pure light. This treatment will run for forty minutes and will end with Mikao Usui's Reiki Crystal of Awakening performing integration Reiki for the last ten minutes of the healing.

Reiki Treatment #9: Mikao Usui's Reiki Crystal of Awakening is sending you a Reiki treatment for success, to release all obstacles to your success and transform them into pure light. This treatment will run for forty minutes and will end with Mikao Usui's Reiki Crystal of Awakening performing integration Reiki for the last ten minutes of the healing.

Reiki Treatment #10: Mikao Usui's Reiki Crystal of Awakening is sending you a Reiki treatment for finding a better job, to activate and open the pathways for either promotion, a raise or an entirely new and better work situation. This treatment will run for forty minutes and will end with Mikao Usui's Reiki Crystal of Awakening performing integration Reiki for the last ten minutes of the healing.

Reiki Treatment #11: Mikao Usui's Reiki Crystal of Awakening is sending you a Reiki treatment for finding a better living situation, to activate and open the pathways for the best possible living situation according to your highest good. This treatment will run for forty minutes and will end with Mikao Usui's Reiki Crystal of Awakening performing integration Reiki for the last ten minutes of the healing.

Reiki Treatment #12: Mikao Usui's Reiki Crystal of Awakening is sending a Reiki treatment to your pet [pet's name] to maintain their well-being according to their highest good. This treatment will run for forty minutes and will end with Mikao Usui's Reiki Crystal of Awakening performing integration Reiki for the last ten minutes of the healing.

Reiki Treatment #13: Mikao Usui's Reiki Crystal of Awakening is sending a Reiki treatment to your car to maintain the car's best functioning according to your highest good. This treatment will run for forty minutes and will end with Mikao Usui's Reiki Crystal of Awakening performing integration Reiki for the last ten minutes of the healing.

As one who often sends Reiki to inanimate objects and machines, and has seen amazing results, I highly recommend this. Obviously, it will not repair a broken window or flat tire, but can help maintain the optimum functioning of an automobile. An addition to this is to ask the Reiki crystal to attune the gas and oil in your car to Reiki, which also contributes to optimal functioning.

Reiki Treatment #14: Mikao Usui's Reiki Crystal of Awakening is sending a Reiki treatment to your computer to maintain its functioning according to the highest good. This treatment will run for forty minutes and will end with Mikao Usui's Reiki Crystal of Awakening performing integration Reiki for the last ten minutes of the healing.

Reiki Treatment #15: Mikao Usui's Reiki Crystal of Awakening is sending a Reiki treatment to your love relationship between you and [name of person] to maintain the highest good. This treatment will run for forty minutes and will end with Mikao Usui's Reiki Crystal of Awakening performing integration Reiki for the last ten minutes of the healing.

Similar to an energy clearing between two people, this treatment requires only the consent of one of the individuals. The treatment activates the energy between both parties for the highest good, and is not a direct treatment to either individual.

Reiki Treatment #16: Mikao Usui's Reiki Crystal of Awakening is sending a Reiki treatment to the work relationship between you and [name of person] to maintain the highest good. This treatment will run for forty minutes and will end with Mikao Usui's Reiki Crystal of Awakening performing integration Reiki for the last ten minutes of the healing.

Same as with any situational or relationship form of Reiki, all that is required is the consent of one of the individuals involved.

Reiki Treatment #17: Mikao Usui's Reiki Crystal of Awakening is sending a Reiki treatment to clear the land surrounding [name the location]. This treatment will run for forty minutes and will end with Mikao Usui's Reiki Crystal of Awakening performing integration Reiki for the last ten minutes of the healing.

Treatments for the land can positively impact relationships, homes, work environments, and more. And, it is important to know and realize that Reiki is not intended only for human beings.

Reiki Treatment #18: Mikao Usui's Reiki Crystal of Awakening is sending a Reiki treatment to clear your day of all energetic obstacles. This treatment will run for forty minutes and will end with Mikao Usui's Reiki Crystal of Awakening performing integration Reiki for the last ten minutes of the healing. (Use at the start of your day, or whenever needed.)

Reiki Treatment #19: Mikao Usui's Reiki Crystal of Awakening is sending a Reiki treatment to clear your ancestral lineage of all energetic obstacles. This treatment will run for forty minutes and will end with Mikao Usui's Reiki Crystal of Awakening performing integration Reiki for the last ten minutes of the healing. (A good treatment to use when things feel stuck and nothing else seems to help.)

Reiki Treatment #20: Mikao Usui's Reiki Crystal of Awakening is sending a Reiki treatment to bring forgiveness into your ancestral lineage for all trespasses against others. This treatment will run for forty minutes and will end with Mikao Usui's Reiki Crystal of Awakening performing integration Reiki for the last ten minutes of the healing. (Another good treatment to use when things feel stuck and nothing else seems to help.)

Reiki Treatment #21: Mikao Usui's Reiki Crystal of Awakening is sending a Reiki Feng Shui treatment to bring energetic balance and Divine order into [name the room being treated]. This treatment will run for ten minutes and will end with Mikao Usui's Reiki Crystal of Awakening performing integration Reiki for the last two minutes of the healing.

Reiki Treatment #22: Mikao Usui's Reiki Crystal of Awakening is sending you a Reiki treatment to deepen your relationship with the Divine. This treatment will run for twenty minutes and will end with Mikao Usui's Reiki Crystal of Awakening performing integration Reiki for the last five minutes of the healing.

Reiki Treatment #23: Mikao Usui's Reiki Crystal of Awakening is sending you a Reiki treatment to deepen your relationship with the angelic realm. This treatment will run for twenty minutes and will end with Mikao Usui's Reiki Crystal of Awakening performing integration Reiki for the last five minutes of the healing.

Reiki Treatment #24: Mikao Usui's Reiki Crystal of Awakening is sending you a Reiki treatment to deepen your relationship with your spirit guides. This treatment will run for twenty minutes and will end with Mikao Usui's Reiki Crystal of Awakening performing integration Reiki for the last five minutes of the healing.

Reiki Treatment #25: Mikao Usui's Reiki Crystal of Awakening is sending you a Reiki treatment to deepen your relationship with the fairy realm. This treatment will run for twenty minutes and will end with Mikao Usui's Reiki Crystal of Awakening performing integration Reiki for the last five minutes of the healing.

Reiki Treatment #26: Mikao Usui's Reiki Crystal of Awakening is sending you a Reiki treatment to deepen your relationship with all life. This treatment will run for twenty minutes and will end with Mikao Usui's Reiki Crystal of Awakening performing integration Reiki for the last five minutes of the healing.

Reiki Treatment #27: Mikao Usui's Reiki Crystal of Awakening is sending you a Reiki treatment to deepen your relationship with yourself. This treatment will run for twenty minutes and will end with Mikao Usui's Reiki Crystal of Awakening performing integration Reiki for the last five minutes of the healing.

Reiki Treatment #28: Mikao Usui's Reiki Crystal of Awakening is sending a deeply relaxing Reiki treatment to you for releasing stress. This treatment will run for twenty minutes and will end with Mikao Usui's Reiki Crystal of Awakening performing integration Reiki for the last five minutes of the healing.

Reiki Treatment #29: Mikao Usui's Reiki Crystal of Awakening is sending you a Reiki treatment to clear your gates of consciousness of all negative energy and negative attachments. This treatment will run for twenty minutes and will end with Mikao Usui's Reiki Crystal of Awakening performing integration Reiki for the last five minutes of the healing.

The gates of consciousness are two acupressure points at the base of the skull. Often, negative energy can collect here. Hence the saying that someone who is negative *can be a pain in the neck*, because the negative energy they create for others can actually accumulate where the top of the neck meets the base of the skull. This treatment when done on a regular basis can help keep your mind clear, and allow you to be less likely to become stressed.

Reiki Treatment #30: Mikao Usui's Reiki Crystal of Awakening is sending you a Reiki treatment to create harmony in your relationships with others. This treatment will run for twenty minutes and will end with Mikao Usui's Reiki Crystal of Awakening performing integration Reiki for the last five minutes of the healing.

Reiki Treatment #31: Mikao Usui's Reiki Crystal of Awakening is sending you a Reiki treatment to help your gifts and strengths become more recognized and readily seen. This treatment will run for twenty minutes and will end with Mikao Usui's Reiki Crystal of Awakening performing integration Reiki for the last five minutes of the healing.

Reiki Treatment #32: Mikao Usui's Reiki Crystal of Awakening is sending you a Reiki crystal gem treatment to replicate an energy healing using crystals and gemstones. This treatment will run for twenty minutes and will end with Mikao Usui's Reiki Crystal of Awakening performing integration Reiki for the last five minutes of the healing.

This is an adaptation of one of the techniques from another energy healing modality created by my teacher and mentor, Ric Weinman. Since the Reiki crystal is imbued with Divine consciousness, it will run a Reiki energetic signature of the appropriate gemstones and crystals that would be for your highest good at any particular moment. No two treatments of this are exactly the same.

Reiki Treatment #33: Mikao Usui's Reiki Crystal of Awakening is sending you a Reiki herbal treatment to replicate an energy healing using the medicinal property of herbs. This treatment will run for twenty minutes and will end with Mikao Usui's Reiki Crystal of Awakening performing integration Reiki for the last five minutes of the healing. (The concept is similar to Reiki Treatment #32, but focusing on herbs instead of crystals and gemstones.)

Reiki Treatment #34: Mikao Usui's Reiki Crystal of Awakening is sending you a Reiki mantra treatment to replicate an energy healing using healing mantras. This treatment will run for twenty minutes and will end with Mikao Usui's Reiki Crystal of Awakening performing integration Reiki for the last five minutes of the healing.

The concept is also similar to Reiki Treatments #32 & #33, but focusing on mantras since the Reiki crystal is capable of replicating any mantra as a Reiki vibration or light. You can either pick a specific mantra, or allow Mikao Usui's Reiki Crystal of Awakening to do it for you.

Reiki Treatment #35: Mikao Usui's Reiki Crystal of Awakening is sending you a Reiki planetary treatment to replicate an energy healing using the astrological properties of the planets for your highest good. This treatment will run for twenty minutes and will end with Mikao Usui's Reiki Crystal of Awakening performing integration Reiki for the last five minutes of the healing.

The concept is similar to Reiki Treatments #32, #33 & #34, but focusing on the astrological properties of the planets since the Reiki crystal is capable of replicating any such property as a Reiki vibration or light. You can either pick a specific planet, or allow Mikao Usui's Reiki Crystal of Awakening to do it for you.

Reiki Treatment #36: Mikao Usui's Reiki Crystal of Awakening is sending a Reiki Archangel treatment to you to replicate an energy healing using the properties of the Archangels for your highest good. This treatment will run for twenty minutes and will end with Mikao Usui's Reiki Crystal of Awakening performing integration Reiki for the last five minutes of the healing.

Reiki Treatment #37: Mikao Usui's Reiki Crystal of Awakening is sending a Reiki of Christ Consciousness treatment to you to replicate an energy healing using the properties of Christ Consciousness for your highest good. This treatment will run for twenty minutes and will end with Mikao Usui's Reiki Crystal of Awakening performing integration Reiki for the last five minutes of the healing.

Reiki Treatment #38: Mikao Usui's Reiki Crystal of Awakening is sending a Reiki of Buddha Consciousness treatment to you to replicate an energy healing using the properties of Buddha Consciousness for your highest good. This treatment will run for twenty minutes and will end with Mikao Usui's Reiki Crystal of Awakening performing integration Reiki for the last five minutes of the healing.

Reiki Treatment #39: Mikao Usui's Reiki Crystal of Awakening is sending a Reiki gender equity treatment to you for your highest good. This treatment will run for forty minutes and will end with Mikao Usui's Reiki Crystal of Awakening performing integration Reiki for the last ten minutes of the healing.

The purpose of this treatment is to assist you in releasing any gender bias consciousness in your energy system that is obstructing your highest good. Social programming, such as boys shouldn't cry or girls shouldn't be strong, can often be obstructions to our true path or calling in life, and can limit our most full expression as human beings.

Reiki Treatment #40: Mikao Usui's Reiki Crystal of Awakening is sending a Reiki racial equity treatment to you for your highest good. This treatment will run for forty minutes and will end with Mikao Usui's Reiki Crystal of Awakening performing integration Reiki for the last ten minutes of the healing.

The purpose of this treatment is to assist you in releasing any racial bias consciousness in your energy system which may be inherited from your ancestors that is obstructing your most open development as a human being. Although some energy healers refuse to address issues of racism, often using half-witted interpretations of karma as an excuse for turning a blind eye to social injustice, my own path as an energy healer has shown me that Reiki can address and heal all of our deepest wounds, even wounds that are socially ingrained and based on race, gender and economic status.

Reiki Treatment #41: Mikao Usui's Reiki Crystal of Awakening is sending a Reiki psychic hot tub treatment to you for your highest good. This treatment will run for twenty minutes and will end with Mikao Usui's Reiki Crystal of Awakening performing integration Reiki for the last five minutes of the healing.

As a student of Remote Viewing, there is a place in the cosmos that some Remote Viewers call the psychic hot tub. It is actually a stream of cosmic string that flows through the universe as if it were the circulatory system of the cosmos. When viewed in a remote viewing session, it has a deeply relaxing or almost euphoric sensation to it. Over the years, I have found that sensation can be replicated as a Reiki treatment.

Reiki Treatment #42: Mikao Usui's Reiki Crystal of Awakening is sending a Reiki of the Holy Grail treatment to you for your highest good. This treatment will run for twenty minutes and will end with Mikao Usui's Reiki Crystal of Awakening performing integration Reiki for the last five minutes of the healing.

The Holy Grail, whether or not it ever existed in this dimension, does exist in other realms simply from the power of the legends surrounding this mythical cup. It holds a power of deep restorative healing, and this power can be replicated as a form of Reiki.

Reiki Treatment #43: Mikao Usui's Reiki Crystal of Awakening is sending a Reiki of the Paramatman Light treatment to you for your highest good. This treatment will run for twenty minutes and will end with Mikao Usui's Reiki Crystal of Awakening performing integration Reiki for the last five minutes of the healing.

The Paramatman Light is a Divine energy given out as darshan by Mother Meera, who some consider an incarnation of the Divine Mother. Although the Paramatman Light cannot be accessed in its pure form through this Reiki technique, the Reiki vibration of this light is still healing, and has profound spiritual benefits.

Reiki Treatment #44: Mikao Usui's Reiki Crystal of Awakening is sending a Reiki of the Eighth-Dimensional Crystal of

Nothingness treatment to you for your highest good. This treatment will run for twenty minutes and will end with Mikao Usui's Reiki Crystal of Awakening performing integration Reiki for the last five minutes of the healing.

The Eighth-Dimensional Crystal of Nothingness is an energetic place of boundless consciousness beyond form or limits. It is a tool of the Magical Awakening energy healing system, but can also be replicated as a vibration of Reiki light.

Reiki Treatment #45: Mikao Usui's Reiki Crystal of Awakening is sending a Reiki of whale songs treatment to you for your highest good. This treatment will run for twenty minutes and will end with Mikao Usui's Reiki Crystal of Awakening performing integration Reiki for the last five minutes of the healing.

Whales are known among many shamanic traditions for their deep empathy with all life, and their songs hold great healing power. Their songs can be replicated as a form of Reiki.

Reiki Treatment #46: Mikao Usui's Reiki Crystal of Awakening is sending a Reiki of the Star of David treatment to you for your highest good. This treatment will run for twenty minutes and will end with Mikao Usui's Reiki Crystal of Awakening performing integration Reiki for the last five minutes of the healing.

Reiki Treatment #47: Mikao Usui's Reiki Crystal of Awakening is sending a Reiki of the Kabbalistic Lightning Path treatment to you for your highest good. This treatment will run for twenty minutes and will end with Mikao Usui's Reiki Crystal of Awakening performing integration Reiki for the last five minutes of the healing.

In the Jewish mystical path of Kabbalah, the Lightning Path very efficiently invokes the presence of the Divine down into the world of form through chanting various Hebrew names of God.

Reiki Treatment #48: Mikao Usui's Reiki Crystal of Awakening is sending a Reiki of the Diamond Sutra treatment to you for your highest good. This treatment will run for twenty minutes and will end with Mikao Usui's Reiki Crystal of Awakening performing integration Reiki for the last five minutes of the healing.

The Diamond Sutra is a sacred Buddhist text which when replicated as a form of Reiki can gracefully open the human heart to its mutually self-aware connection with all other sentient beings.

Reiki Treatment #49: Mikao Usui's Reiki Crystal of Awakening is sending a Reiki of Divine Consciousness treatment to you for dissolving the veil of Maya. This treatment will run for twenty minutes and will end with Mikao Usui's Reiki Crystal of Awakening performing integration Reiki for the last five minutes of the healing.

The veil of Maya is an energetic layering of illusion which keeps us believing we are somehow separate from the Divine. This treatment will work only for those who are already ripe to be spiritually awakened.

Reiki Treatment #50: Mikao Usui's Reiki Crystal of Awakening is sending an eighth-dimensional Reiki treatment to you to clear the root causes of suffering. This treatment will run for twenty minutes and will end with Mikao Usui's Reiki Crystal of Awakening performing integration Reiki for the last ten minutes of the healing.

Reiki Treatment #51: Mikao Usui's Reiki Crystal of Awakening is sending a Reiki treatment to you for Divine protection. This treatment will run for twenty minutes and will end with Mikao Usui's Reiki Crystal of Awakening performing integration Reiki for the last five minutes of the healing.

Reiki Treatment #52: Mikao Usui's Reiki Crystal of Awakening is sending Reiki to heal all shame from your psyche for the next twenty minutes and will end with Mikao Usui's Reiki Crystal of Awakening performing integration Reiki for the last five minutes of the healing.

Reiki Treatment #53: Mikao Usui's Reiki Crystal of Awakening is sending Reiki to heal all fear from your psyche for the next twenty minutes and will end with Mikao Usui's Reiki Crystal of Awakening performing integration Reiki for the last five minutes of the healing.

Reiki Treatment #54: Mikao Usui's Reiki Crystal of Awakening is sending Reiki to heal all confusion from your psyche for the next twenty minutes and will end with Mikao Usui's Reiki Crystal of Awakening performing integration Reiki for the last five minutes of the healing.

Reiki Treatment #55: Mikao Usui's Reiki Crystal of Awakening is sending Reiki to heal all indecision in your psyche for the next twenty minutes and will end with Mikao Usui's Reiki Crystal of Awakening performing integration Reiki for the last five minutes of the healing.

Reiki Treatment #56: Mikao Usui's Reiki Crystal of Awakening is sending Reiki to release trauma from your psyche for the next twenty minutes and will end with Mikao Usui's Reiki Crystal of Awakening performing integration Reiki for the last five minutes of the healing.

Reiki Treatment #57: Mikao Usui's Reiki Crystal of Awakening is sending Reiki to you to heal all unresolved anger issues for the next twenty minutes and will end with Mikao Usui's Reiki Crystal of Awakening performing integration Reiki for the last five minutes of the healing.

Reiki Treatment #58: Mikao Usui's Reiki Crystal of Awakening is sending Reiki to you to allow joy to arise in your psyche for the next twenty minutes, and will end with Mikao Usui's Reiki Crystal of Awakening performing integration Reiki for the last five minutes of the healing.

Reiki Treatment #59: Mikao Usui's Reiki Crystal of Awakening is sending Reiki to you to allow freedom to arise in your psyche for the next twenty minutes, and will end with Mikao Usui's Reiki Crystal of Awakening performing integration Reiki for the last five minutes of the healing.

Reiki Treatment #60: Mikao Usui's Reiki Crystal of Awakening is sending Reiki to you to allow a deep sense of Divine mystery to arise in your psyche for the next twenty minutes, and will end with Mikao Usui's Reiki Crystal of Awakening performing integration Reiki for the last five minutes of the healing.

Reiki Treatment #61: Mikao Usui's Reiki Crystal of Awakening is sending Reiki to you to allow all repressed grief to arise and be healed in your psyche for the next thirty minutes. This treatment will end with Mikao Usui's Reiki Crystal of Awakening performing integration Reiki for the last seven minutes of the healing.

Reiki Treatment #62: Mikao Usui's Reiki Crystal of Awakening is sending Reiki to you to repattern your psyche to embrace your highest purpose for the next thirty minutes. This treatment will end with Mikao Usui's Reiki Crystal of Awakening performing integration Reiki for the last seven minutes of the healing.

Reiki Treatment #63: Mikao Usui's Reiki Crystal of Awakening is sending Reiki for the next thirty minutes to you to repattern your psyche to see the best possible options in your life. This treatment will end with Mikao Usui's Reiki Crystal of Awakening performing integration Reiki for the last seven minutes of the healing.

Reiki Treatment #64: Mikao Usui's Reiki Crystal of Awakening is sending Reiki for the next thirty minutes to you to repattern your psyche to awaken your talents. This treatment will end with Mikao Usui's Reiki Crystal of Awakening performing integration Reiki for the last seven minutes of the healing.

Reiki Treatment #65: Mikao Usui's Reiki Crystal of Awakening is sending Reiki for the next thirty minutes to you to repattern your psyche to know what is in your best interest. This treatment will end with Mikao Usui's Reiki Crystal of Awakening performing integration Reiki for the last seven minutes of the healing.

Reiki Treatment #66: Mikao Usui's Reiki Crystal of Awakening is sending Reiki for the next thirty minutes to you to repattern your psyche to know thyself. This treatment will end with Mikao Usui's Reiki Crystal of Awakening performing integration Reiki for the last seven minutes of the healing.

Reiki Treatment #67: Mikao Usui's Reiki Crystal of Awakening is sending Reiki for the next thirty minutes to you to repattern your psyche to accept the things you cannot change. This treatment will end with Mikao Usui's Reiki Crystal of Awakening performing integration Reiki for the last seven minutes of the healing.

Reiki Treatment #68: Mikao Usui's Reiki Crystal of Awakening is sending Reiki for the next thirty minutes to you to repattern your psyche to accept and know Divine love. This treatment will end with Mikao Usui's Reiki Crystal of Awakening performing integration Reiki for the last seven minutes of the healing.

Reiki Treatment #69: Mikao Usui's Reiki Crystal of Awakening is sending Reiki for the next thirty minutes to you to repattern your psyche for self-love. This treatment will end with Mikao Usui's Reiki Crystal of Awakening performing integration Reiki for the last seven minutes of the healing.

Reiki Treatment #70: Mikao Usui's Reiki Crystal of Awakening is sending Reiki for the next thirty minutes to you to repattern your psyche to have compassion for others and yourself. This treatment will end with Mikao Usui's Reiki Crystal of Awakening performing integration Reiki for the last seven minutes of the healing.

Reiki Treatment #71: Mikao Usui's Reiki Crystal of Awakening is sending Reiki for the next ten minutes to you to energize your entire body and energy system. (This treatment is designed simply to give you more energy, and does not require any integration forms of Reiki light.)

Reiki Treatment #72: Mikao Usui's Reiki Crystal of Awakening is sending Reiki for the next ten minutes to clear you from all unhealthy energy, and unhealthy programming from watching negative television. (This treatment is designed simply to clear you from violent or negative images, and negative stereotypes, often found on television and does not require any integration forms of Reiki light.)

Reiki Treatment #73: Mikao Usui's Reiki Crystal of Awakening is sending the Reiki of God's eternal smile to you for the next ten minutes. :) Nothing to integrate, just laugh and be happy!

Reiki Treatment #74: Mikao Usui's Reiki Crystal of Awakening is sending you a Reiki treatment to deepen your relationship with your Higher Self. This treatment will run for twenty minutes and will end with Mikao Usui's Reiki Crystal of Awakening performing integration Reiki for the last five minutes of the healing.

Reiki Treatment #75: Mikao Usui's Reiki Crystal of Awakening is sending you a Reiki treatment to deepen your relationship with your subconscious mind. This treatment will run for twenty minutes and will end with Mikao Usui's Reiki Crystal of Awakening performing integration Reiki for the last five minutes of the healing.

Reiki Treatment #76: Mikao Usui's Reiki Crystal of Awakening is sending you a Reiki treatment to deepen your relationship with your body. This treatment will run for twenty minutes and will end with Mikao Usui's Reiki Crystal of Awakening performing integration Reiki for the last five minutes of the healing.

Reiki Treatment #77: Mikao Usui's Reiki Crystal of Awakening is sending you a Reiki treatment to deepen your relationship with your children. This treatment will run for twenty minutes and will end with Mikao Usui's Reiki Crystal of Awakening performing integration Reiki for the last five minutes of the healing.

If you do not have biological children you can intend a substitute.

Reiki Treatment #78: Mikao Usui's Reiki Crystal of Awakening is sending you a Reiki treatment to deepen your sense of personal integrity. This treatment will run for twenty minutes and will end with Mikao Usui's Reiki Crystal of Awakening performing integration Reiki for the last five minutes of the healing.

Reiki Treatment #79: Mikao Usui's Reiki Crystal of Awakening is sending you a Reiki treatment to protect and strengthen your personal boundaries. This treatment will run for twenty minutes and will end with Mikao Usui's Reiki Crystal of Awakening performing integration Reiki for the last five minutes of the healing.

Reiki Treatment #80: Mikao Usui's Reiki Crystal of Awakening is sending you a Reiki treatment to deepen your wisdom of how to use Mikao Usui's Reiki Crystal of Awakening. This treatment will run for twenty minutes and will end with Mikao Usui's Reiki Crystal of Awakening performing integration Reiki for the last five minutes of the healing.

Reiki Treatment #81: Mikao Usui's Reiki Crystal of Awakening is sending you a Reiki treatment to deepen your wisdom of how to live in proper alignment with the Earth. This treatment will run for twenty minutes and will end with Mikao Usui's Reiki Crystal of Awakening performing integration Reiki for the last five minutes of the healing.

Reiki Treatment #82: Mikao Usui's Reiki Crystal of Awakening is sending you a Reiki treatment to deepen your wisdom of how to live in proper alignment with the concept of World Peace. This treatment will run for twenty minutes and will end with Mikao Usui's Reiki Crystal of Awakening performing integration Reiki for the last five minutes of the healing.

Reiki Treatment #83: Mikao Usui's Reiki Crystal of Awakening is sending you a Reiki treatment to deepen your wisdom of how to accept your own death. This treatment will run for twenty minutes and will end with Mikao Usui's Reiki Crystal of Awakening performing integration Reiki for the last five minutes of the healing.

Reiki Treatment #84: Mikao Usui's Reiki Crystal of Awakening is sending you a Reiki treatment to deepen your wisdom of how to see yourself as an individual and one with all existence simultaneously. This treatment will run for twenty minutes and will end with Mikao Usui's Reiki Crystal of Awakening performing integration Reiki for the last five minutes of the healing.

Reiki Treatment #85: Mikao Usui's Reiki Crystal of Awakening is sending you a Reiki treatment to deepen your wisdom of how to live fully in the present moment. This treatment will run for twenty minutes and will end with Mikao Usui's Reiki Crystal of Awakening performing integration Reiki for the last five minutes of the healing.

Reiki Treatment #86: Mikao Usui's Reiki Crystal of Awakening is sending you a Reiki treatment to deepen your wisdom of how to best serve the greater good. This treatment will run for twenty minutes and will end with Mikao Usui's Reiki Crystal of Awakening performing integration Reiki for the last five minutes of the healing.

Reiki Treatment #87: Mikao Usui's Reiki Crystal of Awakening is sending you a Reiki treatment to deepen your wisdom of how to be most fully alive. This treatment will run for twenty minutes and will end with Mikao Usui's Reiki Crystal of Awakening performing integration Reiki for the last five minutes of the healing.

Reiki Treatment #88: Mikao Usui's Reiki Crystal of Awakening is sending you a Reiki treatment to deepen your wisdom of how live simply and in alignment with Divine grace. This treatment will run for twenty minutes and will end with Mikao Usui's Reiki Crystal of Awakening performing integration Reiki for the last five minutes of the healing.

Chapter 18

Reiki Meditation Menu

There is a difference between sending Reiki for a mental/emotional effect and using Mikao Usui's Reiki Crystal of Awakening for a meditation. In the former, Reiki is being sent, either traditionally or by using the Reiki crystal, to energetically influence your consciousness for the better. Using Reiki in that manner can bring about very positive changes and dramatic shifts in consciousness, at times opening one to an entirely new perspective. But, that is not the same as an actual Reiki meditation with the Reiki crystal. A meditation with the Reiki crystal is when you actually bring your consciousness into the crystal (as shown in Chapter Eight), so that it is touched and influenced by the Divine consciousness that exists within the Reiki crystal. In that instance, Reiki energy is not necessarily flowing from the Reiki crystal into your mind, but Divine consciousness is.

To best understand this, try an experiment with these two options. First, ask the Reiki crystal to send a short Reiki treatment of several minutes to bring your mental body into a peaceful condition. Do this now, and allow yourself to notice what you experience. Very likely, you may sense some tingling or slight sense of pressure in your head, indicating that Reiki is flowing. Also, as the short treatment runs its course, it is most likely that you will feel a sense of calm or inner peace.

Once the treatment has ended, try performing a Reiki meditation to attain the same outcome by intending that your consciousness sink down into the Reiki crystal and then intending that the Reiki crystal bring your consciousness into a peaceful condition. You may want to refer again to the Reiki meditation technique shown at the end of Chapter Eight. Once you have engaged your consciousness with the consciousness that exists within the Reiki crystal a few inches in front of the center of your chest, simply hold that intention that the Reiki crystal is literally pouring Divine consciousness into your mind to bring about the desired outcome of inner peace.

Notice how these two Reiki techniques feel, and how they differ. Both are useful, but each has a different way of engaging with you. In the previous chapter you learned many Reiki treatments that are hardwired into Mikao Usui's Reiki Crystal of Awakening, and which can be activated by name. Now, you will experience various Reiki meditations that can also be activated by name. By you simply naming them, Mikao Usui's Reiki Crystal of Awakening will literally draw your consciousness down into the crystal, and there begin co-creating new thoughts, new insights which are inspired by the Divine consciousness that is imbued into Mikao Usui's Reiki Crystal of Awakening.

The meditations which follow are intended to get you to practice meditating with the Reiki crystal, to deepen your relationship with it and therefore also with the Divine. Again, this crystal is simply an energetic embodiment of Divine grace. So, do not think you are being asked to change your spiritual or religious beliefs. Mikao Usui was a human being, not God. But the energy of Reiki has evolved to a place where it is imbued with this Divine consciousness and is now an embodiment of Divine grace. So, through the Reiki crystal it is possible to commune with the Divine. What name you give to the Divine, or what religion you may follow, is entirely up to you.

To activate the meditation, simply say out loud or through intention which Reiki meditation you would like to experience. For the best clarity, do not activate more than one Reiki meditation at a time. And, know each will end at the most appropriate time. But, if you feel the need to end a meditation before it has come to a natural end, simply ask the Reiki crystal to disengage you from the meditation.

Reiki Meditation #1
Mikao Usui's Reiki Crystal of Awakening is teaching you that which you need to know most at this point in time.

Reiki Meditation #2
Mikao Usui's Reiki Crystal of Awakening is leading your consciousness to the outer spiritual realms with which is it familiar, and beyond.

Reiki Meditation #3
Mikao Usui's Reiki Crystal of Awakening is showing you your true spiritual nature.

Reiki Meditation #4
Mikao Usui's Reiki Crystal of Awakening is merging your consciousness with the consciousness of Gaia.

Reiki Meditation #5
Mikao Usui's Reiki Crystal of Awakening is employing the consciousness of the Divine to reflect your highest potential back to you.

Reiki Meditation #6
Mikao Usui's Reiki Crystal of Awakening is drawing your consciousness to feel the deepest meaning of your life.

Reiki Meditation #7
Mikao Usui's Reiki Crystal of Awakening is teaching you how to forgive someone you would like to forgive.

Reiki Meditation #8
Mikao Usui's Reiki Crystal of Awakening is showing you your limits and how to respect them.

Reiki Meditation #9

Mikao Usui's Reiki Crystal of Awakening is showing you your weaknesses, and how to overcome what weaknesses you can, and accept that which cannot be overcome.

Reiki Meditation #10

Mikao Usui's Reiki Crystal of Awakening is showing you your most important virtues, as well as those you can better aspire to.

Reiki Meditation #11

Mikao Usui's Reiki Crystal of Awakening is bringing your consciousness into absolute stillness.

Reiki Meditation #12

Mikao Usui's Reiki Crystal of Awakening is shedding lust from your consciousness.

Reiki Meditation #13

Mikao Usui's Reiki Crystal of Awakening is shedding wrath from your consciousness.

Reiki Meditation #14

Mikao Usui's Reiki Crystal of Awakening is shedding greed from your consciousness.

Reiki Meditation #15

Mikao Usui's Reiki Crystal of Awakening is shedding hate from your consciousness.

Reiki Meditation #16

Mikao Usui's Reiki Crystal of Awakening is shedding jealousy from your consciousness.

Reiki Meditation #17
Mikao Usui's Reiki Crystal of Awakening is shedding pride from your consciousness.

Reiki Meditation #18
Mikao Usui's Reiki Crystal of Awakening is shedding arrogance from your consciousness.

Reiki Meditation #19
Mikao Usui's Reiki Crystal of Awakening is shedding vanity from your consciousness.

Reiki Meditation #20
Mikao Usui's Reiki Crystal of Awakening is shedding wastefulness from your consciousness.

Reiki Meditation #21
Mikao Usui's Reiki Crystal of Awakening is shedding ingratitude from your consciousness.

Reiki Meditation #22
Mikao Usui's Reiki Crystal of Awakening is activating courage in your consciousness.

Reiki Meditation #23
Mikao Usui's Reiki Crystal of Awakening is activating faith in your consciousness.

Reiki Meditation #24
Mikao Usui's Reiki Crystal of Awakening is activating hope in your consciousness.

Reiki Meditation #25
Mikao Usui's Reiki Crystal of Awakening is activating charity in

your consciousness.

Reiki Meditation #26
Mikao Usui's Reiki Crystal of Awakening is activating kindness in your consciousness.

Reiki Meditation #27
Mikao Usui's Reiki Crystal of Awakening is activating honesty in your consciousness.

Reiki Meditation #28
Mikao Usui's Reiki Crystal of Awakening is activating love in your consciousness.

Reiki Meditation #29
Mikao Usui's Reiki Crystal of Awakening is activating gratitude in your consciousness.

Reiki Meditation #30
Mikao Usui's Reiki Crystal of Awakening is activating ecstasy in your consciousness.

Reiki Meditation #31
Mikao Usui's Reiki Crystal of Awakening is activating an awareness of the Divine in your consciousness.

Reiki Meditation #32
Mikao Usui's Reiki Crystal of Awakening is activating a love for the Divine in your consciousness.

Reiki Meditation #33
Mikao Usui's Reiki Crystal of Awakening is activating the golden rule in your consciousness.

Reiki Meditation #34
Mikao Usui's Reiki Crystal of Awakening is activating Oneness in your consciousness.

Reiki Meditation #35
Mikao Usui's Reiki Crystal of Awakening is activating the four noble truths of Buddhism in your consciousness.

Reiki Meditation #36
Mikao Usui's Reiki Crystal of Awakening is activating the 23rd Psalm in your consciousness.

Reiki Meditation #37
Mikao Usui's Reiki Crystal of Awakening is activating the Prayer of Saint Francis in your consciousness.

Reiki Meditation #38
Mikao Usui's Reiki Crystal of Awakening is activating Divine laughter in your consciousness.

Reiki Meditation #39
Mikao Usui's Reiki Crystal of Awakening is activating humility in your consciousness.

Reiki Meditation #40
Mikao Usui's Reiki Crystal of Awakening is showing you your own ego in your consciousness.

Reiki Meditation #41
Mikao Usui's Reiki Crystal of Awakening is blowing the wind of Divine Grace through your consciousness.

Reiki Meditation #42
Mikao Usui's Reiki Crystal of Awakening is radiating Divine love

for you in your consciousness.

Reiki Meditation #43

Mikao Usui's Reiki Crystal of Awakening is revealing in your consciousness that which you were before birth.

Reiki Meditation #44

Mikao Usui's Reiki Crystal of Awakening is revealing in your consciousness that which you will be after death.

Chapter 19

Reiki Affirmations

The affirmations below are charged with Reiki in such a way that each affirmation is simultaneously sending you energy while also guiding your consciousness into a desired place of being. One may think of it as a merging of a mini Reiki treatment and a mini Reiki meditation simultaneously. Each Reiki affirmation is designed to work on anyone, whether or not they happen to be a Reiki practitioner, and even if they have not done the work of the previous chapters of this book. These affirmations can be shared with friends and family as a gentle way to introduce them to this work, or simply as a way to widen the circle of Reiki light deeper into the world.

To work with each affirmation, say the entire affirmation out loud. As you do, Reiki is being generated from the affirmation itself to flow into your consciousness. Also, the words themselves are each empowered with Mikao Usui's Reiki Crystal of Awakening, and have the ability to draw your consciousness into an interactive meditation. The combination of these two, the energy healing and interactive meditation, can be quite powerful. Each affirmation is designed to go deeper the more you repeat it at any given time.

Reiki Affirmation #1
I deeply love and appreciate myself. I deeply love and appreciate myself. I deeply love and appreciate myself.

Reiki Affirmation #2
I am releasing all negative thought patterns and replacing them with love and light. I am releasing all negative thought patterns and replacing them with love and light. I am releasing all

negative thought patterns and replacing them with love and light.

Reiki Affirmation #3

I am open to freedom and new possibilities. I am open to freedom and new possibilities. I am open to freedom and new possibilities.

Reiki Affirmation #4

I am clearing my chakras of all psychic debris and filling each chakra with Divine light. I am clearing my chakras of all psychic debris and filling each chakra with Divine light. I am clearing my chakras of all psychic debris and filling each chakra with Divine light.

Reiki Affirmation #5

I am vibrant, healthy and passionately alive. I am vibrant, healthy and passionately alive. I am vibrant, healthy and passionately alive.

Reiki Affirmation #6

I am financially abundant and have all that I need. I am financially abundant and have all that I need. I am financially abundant and have all that I need.

Reiki Affirmation #7

I am lucky and fortunate in all that I do. I am lucky and fortunate in all that I do. I am lucky and fortunate in all that I do.

Reiki Affirmation #8

I am sexy, wise and illuminated. I am sexy, wise and illuminated. I am sexy, wise and illuminated.

Reiki Affirmation #9
I am driven and accomplish my goals. I am driven and accomplish my goals. I am driven and accomplish my goals.

Reiki Affirmation #10
I am nurturing of myself and others. I am nurturing of myself and others. I am nurturing of myself and others.

Reiki Affirmation #11
I am a spiritual warrior who is fair and just. I am a spiritual warrior who is fair and just. I am a spiritual warrior who is fair and just.

Reiki Affirmation #12
I am a playful and well-integrated human being. I am a playful and well-integrated human being. I am a playful and well-integrated human being.

Reiki Affirmation #13
I am open to Divine guidance and inspiration. I am open to Divine guidance and inspiration. I am open to Divine guidance and inspiration.

Reiki Affirmation #14
I am joyful and know what I want. I am joyful and know what I want. I am joyful and know what I want.

Reiki Affirmation #15
I am mentally alert and conscious of all that I need to know. I am mentally alert and conscious of all that I need to know. I am mentally alert and conscious of all that I need to know.

Reiki Affirmation #16
I am Divinely protected and perfectly safe. I am Divinely

protected and perfectly safe. I am Divinely protected and perfectly safe.

Reiki Affirmation #17

I am harmonious, trustworthy and loyal. I am harmonious, trustworthy and loyal. I am harmonious, trustworthy and loyal.

Reiki Affirmation #18

I express right discernment, and harmonize my rhythm with the rhythm of the world. I express right discernment, and harmonize my rhythm with the rhythm of the world. I express right discernment, and harmonize my rhythm with the rhythm of the world.

Reiki Affirmation #19

I am a beautiful soul. I am a beautiful soul. I am a beautiful soul.

Reiki Affirmation #20

I am experiencing the emptiness of who I am before and after I came into this world of form. I am experiencing the emptiness of who I am before and after I came into this world of form. I am experiencing the emptiness of who I am before and after I came into this world of form.

Reiki Affirmation #21

I am one and at peace with all that is. I am one and at peace with all that is. I am one and at peace with all that is.

Reiki Affirmation #22

I am free and integrated within that which I call family and home. I am free and integrated within that which I call family and home. I am free and integrated within that which I call family and home.

Chapter 20

Ten Laws of Reiki

I have been studying the energy of Reiki for over two decades, not simply trusting in what my teachers have told me but using experiments with the energy itself to teach me of what was possible. My experiments over the years have shown me ten laws of Reiki. These laws are not intended to limit the possibilities, but to give structure to what one can do with Reiki. These ten laws of Reiki as I see them are:

1   Reiki is guided by Divine intelligence and always works for the highest good.
2   Reiki is a living and evolving system, and cannot be defined only by its history.
3   Anything human, animal, plant, mineral, animate or inanimate, can be attuned to Reiki energy.
4   Reiki energy will flow forth from anything which has been attuned to Reiki.
5   Reiki can be molded into shapes, elemental forces, words, colors, symbols, essentially anything that exists, and then infused into the body for a deeper healing, using Mikao Usui's Reiki Crystal of Awakening (or the Higher Self Reiki techniques explored in my other books).
6   The most important voice a Reiki student needs to listen to is the voice of the energy itself.
7   Those who surrender to listening to Reiki energy will be shown new techniques and abilities as the Reiki system continues to evolve.
8   Sending Reiki through time and space can happen because Reiki and the source of all Reiki are beyond both time and space. In other words, Reiki is more than just

the collective sum of life force energy created by living things, but instead comes from a higher realm than the one we live in.

9 Reiki does not discriminate between those who can feel the energy and those who cannot.

10 As long as one respects the free will of others to accept or decline a Reiki treatment, the only limit to what one can do with Reiki is the limit of one's own imagination.

My own sense is that these laws have been evident to me for quite some time. But, this is the first time I ever considered writing them out for others. It has been my error to assume these laws as common knowledge among other Reiki masters or most Reiki practitioners. The reason I add them here is because as evolved and as powerful as Mikao Usui's Reiki Crystal of Awakening is, I do not assume it is the end of the road in terms of the evolution of this fabulous energy healing system we call Reiki. In fact, my sense is this is really only the tip of the iceberg. And, as long as we have laws that tell us of these possibilities and the guidelines they function under, we will no longer look blindly to what our teachers have taught us, and instead will learn directly from our experience of the energy itself.

Chapter 21

Reiki Psalms

A psalm is a sacred song or hymn, and although often attributed to the Bible there are psalms in other spiritual traditions as well. The Reiki psalms below are intended to elicit a deeper sense of communion with the Divine. They function similarly to Reiki affirmations, but are deeper energetically and more eloquent. Simply reading the Reiki psalm engages you with an energetic Reiki blessing contained inside of each psalm, though speaking each out loud will engage you with an even deeper layer of the Reiki blessing. Each of the Reiki psalms is intended not as a replacement for your own spiritual tradition, but to help access a deeper energetic form of the Divine grace that Reiki is.

Reiki Psalm 1

Bless the world as seen through my eyes
And teach me to listen
Inside every hour is a universe
a place of time
from which I can neither escape nor move
but must wade slowly
captured by grace
exalted to witness that which is beyond my comprehension
I expand eternally with each breath
Yet cannot know what it means to be limitless without end
except in this moment

Reiki Psalm 2

When light becomes word
and word becomes joy
there I am deeply immersed in Divine grace

allowing it to surround my ego
dissolving the me that I was never born to become
but only meant to awaken

Reiki Psalm 3

My wounded heart wishes to be whole
and filled with prophecy of times unlearned
where the gift of love is boundless
and all in every direction is praise for the mad glory of
  existence
There I will see that which is the cure to my ailment
There will I be held and nourished with infinite light
There will I know who I am beyond the self I have imagined
  myself to be

Reiki Psalm 4

Protect me from the angry words of others
And take away all my suffering
Bring peace to my ears
Bring peace to my eyes
Bring peace to my thought
So that I may be reborn into light
So that each whisper of Divine word
is one I can capture and taste
Let me consume this light
and also be consumed by it
Let me ravish the flesh of this light
and be ravished within it
Let me shout love for all beings
and see that love reflected back to me
as it is simultaneously then sent back to them as well
Let me know who I came into this world to be

Reiki Psalm 5

To be in bed with the Divine
and sleep with a nursed pillow
and feel held eternally
why would anyone not desire this
let me end all need for explanation
even to my own mind
let my mind be lost in the thrill of its own emptiness
for that is the only place I can know
A wave of light washes my face
purifying the image of who I send into the world
Another wave of light caresses my heart
telling me there is no need to feel alone
How can I do anything but dance in this place
to empty myself of anything other than ecstasy

Reiki Psalm 6

I am falling through an infinite window in time
and as I fall I know I am falling through everywhere
moving through each kind thought
roaming the ignition of galaxies and stars
eternally grasping with my fingers at the yes of all existence

Reiki Psalm 7

Surrender and give yourself away
Each tower built is created only to be tumbled into a
    gemstone of emptiness
Surround yourself with a simple task
which is to love

Reiki Psalm 8

Some see the light as a business
others as a hierarchy
others still, as not existing at all

yet I see the light as emanating eternally
growing me back into the moment of my destiny
rounding the curve of the latest square
bringing passion to the numbers on an infinite line of digits
solving the mystery before expanding it into a glorious feast
I am light and came from light
I am the food from which I must grow
I am the being which has never been the same in any given
    moment
And yet I try to define myself endlessly
only to round myself amusingly into a ball
like a small child
whistling to the sky as an ant plays and struggles with a blade
    of grass
so tender is the way of knowing

Reiki Psalm 9

Burn yourself like a piece of paper
becoming heat and light
never fearing the ashes of your own illumination

Reiki Psalm 10

Within the avenues of time
excellence becomes a wall
perfect placement of hands
a twisted arrogance of symbols
then, the marketing of everything to stay alive
So grateful am I to be still in this moment
unconcerned with the destiny of others
just to breathe in the light
and feel illuminated
as if there was no one in the universe to worry about
not even myself

Reiki Psalm 11

Implant your thoughts within the Reiki crystal
and let it unwind within you all that needs release
Be as a cosmic star ready to shine your brilliance among the
heavens
Have you ever known a star afraid of its own light?
Or witnessed a galaxy shame itself being too illuminated
Yet we who are human prefer to doubt that light within
To tuck it under ourselves
and let it bleed until the light itself is gone, and only a shadow
exists
Cast off all that you are not willing to be
even the replacement for yourself so well manufactured with
manners and social niceties
be true to the light within
and the light without will shine even brighter than before

Reiki Psalm 12

Unfold wise acres of light
with songs of light
become wisdom
as energy passes
trapping not even the witnessing of your own mind
as these words are written so too do they pull from the intelligence
of Divine mind
Who created this body of language
Where are you being when not thinking of yourself
Become, and the universe will indulge you
Run away, and it will chase after you like a zealot

Reiki Psalm 13

Chase yourself like a dog after its own tail
the bonus of living in a modern world

to update your own image relentlessly
yet with soft hands you can understand the meaning of time
and with soft eyes you can hear the sound of each angel
     singing to God
and with soft legs, you can stand strong never to be pushed
     over
Give your silence to yourself
And know the road to heaven is paved with emptiness

Reiki Psalm 14

Challenges disturb the mind
yet we harness our wisdom from ancient laws
which many are now dormant, lost, forgotten
What new laws can one read that are still ancient
like carrying a prayer uphill inside a bucket of water
waiting to spill it on those you love
Just step forward
let your hands drop
and all will be amazing

Reiki Psalm 15

Enter into the splendid Divine
like tumbling as a child into a pool of water
with laughter and joy
all you ever imagined is still possible
still within reach
just hold the belief
shine your eyes upon your fingertips
and let wishes fly from your mind like butterflies

Reiki Psalm 16

This great fascination with ego and mind
We are all nothing more
than imaginary friends of the Divine

Reiki Psalm 17

Again I am no one
whispering in the light of the Divine
telling myself who I am by the words that I see
going into places I cannot know, yet have felt inside of me
    forever
I am bleeding now
and each drop is a desire to know and be known
to learn and be taught
here in the classroom of Divine mind
I gain all that I need to know
becoming precious as a drop of honey

Reiki Psalm 18

Relax into the plentiful now
where many universes dance simultaneously
each one a precious child of the Divine
like a wheelbarrow of candy displayed through all time
Our hands cannot know which piece is meant for us
where to grasp and let go
of what it is we need to be soft enough
or hard enough
to chew or let our tongues dance lightly
so sweet is this life
I fall deep into the sugar of each moment
knowing I myself will eventually be eaten
like candy for the Divine

Reiki Psalm 19

Numbers tickle my eyes
as if anything can be less than infinite
to swallow the hard digits as real
when the luminous essence behind them is a nectar
unfolding eternally

grasped not by mind, nor even heart
but in the act of ever emptying
there I can stand tall
almost naked to the world
knowing myself
both human and beyond

Reiki Psalm 20

Sweeter than I ever came to be
joined by the mystery of now
and a chatter as wise as the loose lips of a stranger
I dance with each moment
and breathe sighs upon the canvass of the sky
deliver this now
Usui has given me a gift far beyond my ability to comprehend

Reiki Psalm 21

Beloved inner being
where is the crest of your knowledge
delightful and loud
twisting like a lover inside a cloud
I choose not to see myself in the mirror
just wondering if the power of reflection itself
is enough
to keep measuring the eyes of time

Reiki Psalm 22

I became a rainbow illuminated at night
how noble for the sun's rays to find me there
twisting through the atmosphere
to brighten my world from the inside out
seeing golden speeches of color dance through me and beyond

Reiki Psalm 23

Below myself I escape
into the dust
of who I am
and there am blown across the landscape of destiny
so curious to be launched like a ship full of ceremony and
    praise
awake to each storm, the greatest of which is always inside
my hands light up like lamps
filled with an eternal oil
I am alive
always seeking to be yes and yes and over again
tumbling with each wave of light
being rediscovered at my core

Reiki Psalm 24

My eyes have awakened
seeing only that which is
aspiring to be love
Behind my face
no one resides
and inside my ears
there is only a mantra of Divine names
Explode with me into a speckle of eternal laughter
Each syllable a crown made of gold

Reiki Psalm 25

Let go of all explanation
There is no mind to convince
No place that is capable of regulating life
Only mystery unfolding
To cherish each footstep
all by itself
the footstep cherishing the body as well

Go into the quietly opening spaces
and there stand
until no sound is capable of manifesting
not even a prayer
for prayers themselves can even be a distraction at times
Be a prayer
rather than reciting one

Reiki Psalm 26

I roll about inside infinity
dragging my mind in my hands
if only I could let it go
like a flower
to be something on its own
Split open my thoughts
to spill light into each one
and let it radiate like a galaxy
spinning open in the hand of the Divine

Reiki Psalm 27

Bliss is the name of love
even when tired
even when lost
but to smile in those moments
when tears are almost raining from your eyes
that is the precious way of being
the rotunda of your consciousness echoing out the brightest
    star
such Divine language we speak
Do not allow yourself to be mute
when conversing of love

Reiki Psalm 28

Be alone in the winter of time

There you will find all that is needed
to witness each star witnessing you
then to inhale each band of starlight
Fear nothing
when nothing
is fearful
Be loved
when love
is being you
note the answers
most given
by birds, animals and strangers
they usually speak the truth

Reiki Psalm 29

Today angels scrubbed my face with joy
and instead of taking them for granted
I worshipped the light they are made of
I smoked their feathers to intoxicate my mind with Divine
     ecstatic madness
I reveled in their dances, their songs to all creation
and then I imagined what it must mean for an angel to fly
to fly and yet be made of nothing but light
how swell an offering each act of ascension must be
Dismantling the sub-rhythms
the turbulent decisions
I burst open into pure light
and shined like an arch angel gone super nova

Reiki Psalm 30

There is no language beyond
no ancient script that can illuminate
the disjointed aspects of humanity
until every hair sings the right song

and each elbow is tucked away and ready
to be the partner in a universal dance
How can one fail when dancing arm linked with brother or
    sister
How can we give mercy to our friends
and not discuss their failings in their absence
How can we know the greatest service to ourselves
is to serve the need of everyone

Reiki Psalm 31

Infinity cast out like dice
rolling to scrub my eyes
until the game is won
I sing the song of infinity
and dance along the eternal kiss

Reiki Psalm 32

Love is an orchard of strangers
each holding an apple
filled with the brightest light imaginable
if only we will breathe

Reiki Psalm 33

In this moment
radiate your heart in the direction of love
make this your compass
the true north
by which every action is measured
and every thought is known
dance with your feet wanting to turn the planet
each time they touch the earth
these are simple words to live by
just know them

Chapter 22

Time Released Reiki Treatments & Your Daily Practice

One of the beautiful aspects of Mikao Usui's Reiki Crystal of Awakening is the ability to program an entire series of Reiki treatments ahead of time to run at specific junctures during your day. You can do this when waking up in the morning to send Reiki to your entire day, to an important meeting, to yourself at a time when you may feel stressed, and for deeper personal healing. This ability makes it easy for you to integrate Reiki into all aspects of your life.

To do this, all you need to do is take several minutes when you wake up in the morning to intentionally program a series of Reiki time released treatments to run during your day. Simply say out loud the series of treatments you wish for the crystal to run, and also specify when you want each treatment to begin. While specifying when you want each treatment to begin, know that you can link that start time of the treatment to either a specific time or a specific action. For example, if you know you will want some Reiki when you get home from work but are not exactly sure what time that will be, simply program into the crystal that it send the treatment to you once you arrive home from work. Create a list of Reiki treatments or Reiki meditations you would like to receive during the day. Such a list may look like the sample list below.

7 am – Start day with Reiki meditation #5 for five minutes.
7:30 am – Send Reiki to clear my breakfast of all negative energy and optimize the food for my body.
8 am – Send a ten-minute treatment to my day at work and to optimize the workplace.

12 noon – Send a Reiki treatment to clear my lunch of all negative energy and optimize the food for my body.

6 pm – Send Reiki treatment #41 (psychic hot tub treatment) to myself when I get home from work.

7 pm – Send a Reiki treatment to clear my dinner of all negative energy and optimize the food for my body.

11 pm – Send myself Reiki treatment #6.

Once you have created the list of Reiki treatments you want for the day, simply program that list into Mikao Usui's Reiki Crystal of Awakening either through thought, visualization, or simply speaking out loud that you would like the Reiki crystal to send you Reiki treatments throughout your day according to the list.

You can also add Reiki affirmations and Reiki psalms to your daily practice, which will deepen the overall effect. However, since Reiki affirmations and Reiki psalms are intended to be spoken and/or read, they cannot be programmed into the Reiki crystal the way treatments and meditations can. Still, you can integrate them quite easily into a daily routine by speaking your list to the Reiki crystal in the morning, and then weaving in Reiki affirmations during the day, and reading a Reiki psalm of two before you go to bed in the evening. The purpose of all of this is simply to bring as much of this Divine light into your life as possible.

Chapter 23

Reiki Holograms, Reiki Magical Devices and Other Sacred Games

My book *Reiki for Spiritual Healing* explores the concepts of Reiki holograms and Reiki magical devices in depth, as well as other concepts such as Reiki color grids. Such concepts were entirely new to Reiki when the book was released, and still to this day are very cutting edge in the possible options they provide to a Reiki healer. The concept behind them primarily is that Reiki as a flow of energy is just one aspect of the energy, and that Reiki is also a malleable form of spiritual light that can be molded as if it were a kind of spiritual clay. Originally, the only way I knew how to do this was by working in collaboration with my Higher Self, a part of the human energetic body that according to many cultures, including that of ancient Egyptians and Hawaiian shamans, exists beyond time and space. The process explained in my book *Reiki for Spiritual Healing* is one I still use, but I realized over time that some found it too complex or cumbersome to understand. Those who did understand the process loved it, but those who did not seemed to be alienated by it.

Thanks to the Divine intelligence which exists inside of Mikao Usui's Reiki Crystal of Awakening, it is now possible to invoke Reiki holograms and Reiki magical devices simply by asking Mikao Usui's Reiki Crystal to do so. Although in some of the treatments already explained in previous chapters, it is very likely that Mikao Usui's Reiki Crystal of Awakening is already incorporating these Reiki techniques, only that you may not be consciously aware of it. That is because Mikao Usui's Reiki Crystal of Awakening is accessing every Reiki technique ever developed to manifest the desired goal of any specific treatment you request. For that reason, I did not originally intend on including in this book information about Reiki holograms, Reiki magical devices, and other sacred ways that Reiki can be manifested, simply because the Reiki crystal was always going to do this with or without your request as long it was for your highest good.

Yet one of the most important aspects of my Reiki research has been that the Divine, or whatever name you wish to give for the Supreme Being and Creator, enjoys us being childlike and playful, as if we are magical children who can play with the Divine. Often, when teaching Reiki and other energy healing modalities I will encourage my students to play, to discover, to move beyond fear and limitations and know that they can do no harm when playing with Reiki because their playmate in this realm is actually the ever compassionate and ever healing Divine. So, I include this information here about Reiki holograms, Reiki magical devices and other sacred ways of *playing* with Reiki energy, not because they can improve on the most perfect Reiki treatment that will always be sent by Mikao Usui's Reiki Crystal of Awakening, which is already accessing these techniques without you specifying it to do so. But I add this information instead because these are wonderful ways to literally play with the Divine (who is known as God, Goddess and myriad other names).

So, let your inner kid come out and play! And these are the energy toys you get to play with:

A *Reiki hologram* is simply an energetic replication of anything that exists, made out of Reiki light. You can create a Reiki hologram of a rock, a crystal, a hat, a mythological being and more.

A *Reiki magical device* is actually just a very specific type of Reiki hologram, one that is of a spiritual symbol or magical object. So, it contains not only the formation of Reiki light that replicates it, but also is imbued with a Divine essence of the power associated with the given symbol or object. For example, a

Reiki hologram of a halo is a Reiki magical device.

To play with Reiki holograms, Reiki magical devices and more sets forth a conscious interaction between you and the consciousness of the Divine in a way that is not just about asking to be healed or asking to have your life improved. It assumes something instead quite radical for some, especially those few Reiki masters who can be so God awful serious. That assumption is that the Divine actually enjoys our conscious presence, to just be with us. How boring it must be for the Divine to only interact with us when we need something, to have us always asking for help or just giving praise, as if there were no other way we could interact with God. The ability to create Reiki holograms is simply pure playful magic, a kind of magic that relies upon the Divine grace of this amazing energy called Reiki.

Yes, Reiki heals and can change your life in amazing ways. But it is also a medium which can be used to simply and quite literally play with the Divine. This space of Divine play in itself is healing. To try this kind of play, first just create some Reiki holograms. Practice this now by asking Mikao Usui's Reiki Crystal of Awakening to create a Reiki hologram of a butterfly and that it place this Reiki hologram of a butterfly in your right hand. If you are energy sensitive, it is very likely you will sense a presence very similar to a real butterfly appear in your hand. Now, ask Mikao Usui's Reiki Crystal of Awakening to have that Reiki hologram of a butterfly fly around your head. Again, not that you will actually see a butterfly, but it is very likely you will have the sensation of something flying around near your head.

Now, ask Mikao Usui's Reiki Crystal of Awakening to create Reiki holograms of gloves and to place one over each hand. Again, if you are energy sensitive you will very likely have the sensation of wearing invisible gloves made out of Reiki light, but a very discernible presence covering your hands.

Now, ask Mikao Usui's Reiki Crystal of Awakening to create a Reiki magical device of a halo made out of Reiki a few inches above your head. Once you have done this you may feel not just the presence of this circle of Reiki light above your head, but also the opening of your higher mind to a deeper sense of spiritual awareness and wisdom.

The possibilities for creating Reiki holograms and Reiki magical devices are truly endless. They can do no harm, and are simply objects made out of the Divine light called Reiki. I encourage you to play with them, to set your imagination free in a dance with this Divine light.

A last few playful exercises I offer are to ask Mikao Usui's Reiki Crystal of Awakening to create a Reiki hologram of an apple in your right hand. Then, once the Reiki hologram of an apple exists in your hand, take a bite out of it. Notice the Reiki energy still existing in your mouth almost as if you have eaten from a real apple. Then, swallow it and feel the tingling vibration move down into your stomach.

One last exercise is to ask Mikao Usui's Reiki Crystal of Awakening to create a Reiki hologram of this book, and infuse it into each cell of your brain. Remember, since this is Divine consciousness you are playing with do not bother to put rational restrictions on it, for that consciousness is far beyond the world of reason and can make the book as little as it needs to be to fit in each cell of your brain. Then, once you have done this feel the buzzing presence of this book, of all that you have read and learned, as it dances through your consciousness as Reiki.

Be playful! Be joyful! Be imaginative and alive! That is what I sense the Divine wants from us most, something so often missed in the spiritual texts of the world.

The game will always be there for you to play, as long as you are willing to imagine, and willing to playfully engage in this dance of Reiki with the Divine.

The aspect of Mikao Usui's Reiki Crystal of Awakening that exists inside this book is now creating a Reiki hologram of the universe, consolidated down to the size of a pill. If you would like to swallow it, stick out your tongue. Feel the Reiki hologram there, and swallow. Then know there is an entire Reiki universe inside of you. Explore it, and there you will know the mystery, the passion, the beauty of the stars. Let it teach you always of your own Divine eternal magic that you are.

AYNI
BOOKS

"Ayni" is a Quechua word meaning "reciprocity" – sharing, giving and receiving – whatever you give out comes back to you. To be in Ayni is to be in balance, harmony and right relationship with oneself and nature, of which we are all an intrinsic part. Complementary and Alternative approaches to health and well-being essentially follow a holistic model, within which one is given support and encouragement to move towards a state of balance, true health and wholeness, ultimately leading to the awareness of one's unique place in the Universal jigsaw of life – Ayni, in fact.